HOPE AFTER STROKE

HOPE AFTER STROKE
For Caregivers and Survivors
THE HOLISTIC GUIDE TO GETTING YOUR LIFE BACK

ISBN: 978-1-7329538-0-2

While the author has made every effort to provide accurate telephone numbers and Internet addresses at the time of publication, neither the publisher nor the author assumes any responsibility for errors, or for changes that occur after publication.

Publisher: XETROV

Book cover photo credit: Lisa Bragg-Cohen
Book cover design: info.onedesigns@gmail.com

one designs

Illustrations by: Tania Sultana of Web_graphicz
Interior Design: Lazar Kackarovski

HOPE AFTER STROKE

FOR CAREGIVERS AND SURVIVORS

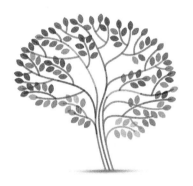

THE HOLISTIC GUIDE TO GETTING YOUR LIFE BACK

by
TSGOYNA TANZMAN, *M.A./CCC SLP*
Speech-Language Pathologist
Life Coach/Master Practitioner NLP

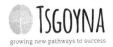

growing new pathways to success

GRAB YOUR FREE BONUS

of

My Recovery Journal & Workbook

A companion to

HOPE AFTER STROKE

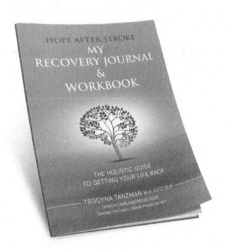

READ THIS FIRST

To jumpstart your recovery and say thanks for downloading
my book, I'd like to gift you with a mini sample of

MY RECOVERY JOURNAL & WORKBOOK

including 21 days of practice

100% FREE

VISIT THIS LINK TO GET STARTED

https://mailchi.mp/af2d2f477a15/free-workbooksample

ACKNOWLEDGMENTS

I f it takes a village to raise a child, it takes a planet to write a book. *Hope After Stroke* was a seed of inspiration planted during a morning meditation, and its roots spread, connecting me to three continents and countless new people across the USA. I am so grateful to those new friends I've met as a result of this project. From the start, I want to acknowledge and thank my parents who long ago passed, but who sat on my desk and guided this writing. I'm especially grateful to my mother, Iris, who introduced me to the world of speech pathology after my grandmother's stroke.

I am appreciative of the knowledge, expertise, and generosity of Dr. Argye Hillis-Trupe, Dr. Jeremy Nobel, Dr. David Levy, Peter G. Levine, Dr. Donna Lundy, Dr. Dolores Malaspina, Dr. Heidi Moawad, and the many other researchers and professionals whose work has informed me. I am grateful to the teams of OTs, PTs, and SWs with whom I've collaborated to help patients find their greatest recovery and who have also offered their invaluable insight and knowledge to this project.

Thank you to my many coaching mentors with whom I've studied and worked: Tony Robbins, Brooke Castillo, Dr. Dawson Church, Derek Rydall, and "Abraham."

I am so thankful for my early believers, supporters, and readers: Lenore, Leslie, Sylvia, and my editor, Jessica, who diligently prodded me to expand upon and clarify stories, descriptions, and research. To Kathleen, Jean, and Valerie, I owe my deepest and most profound appreciation—you opened your hearts and shared candidly about your private bitter and sweet experiences and in so doing, you offer hope to others. Taylor, I am beyond grateful for your enthusiasm, keen vision, and super powers of connection. You are a well of endless knowledge and resources.

In saving the best for last, there are two people without whom this couldn't have happened: My daughter, Zoe, who showered this tiny seed of inspiration with her special brand of magical fertilizer, and most of all my husband, Paul, who not only believed in me and was my biggest promoter, but who supported me by spending hundreds of hours making delicious meals and taking care of the way-too-many-to-recount daily life tasks, just so that I could devote time to writing.

Finally and most especially, I want to thank all of the stroke survivors and families with whom I've worked over the last three decades. I am humbled by and grateful for your trust, allowing me to enter your private lives and be a part of your healing journey. I will always remember you.

TABLE OF CONTENTS

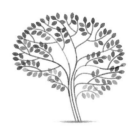

Acknowledgments . . . . *v*

Preface . . . . *xi*

Foreword . . . .*xiii*

Introduction *1*

PART 1   What Happened? *Life in the Hospital*. 7

  1.   *What's in a Name? Get to Know Your Stroke (C)* *9*

  2.   *Advocating for Your Loved One (C)* *19*

  3.   *You are the Center of Your Rehab Team (C&S)* *29*

  4.   *The Secret Sauce of Recovering (C&S)* 47

  5.   *Change your Language, Shape your Life (C&S)*. 59

  6.   *Answering Your Most Pressing "Why" Questions:*
      A Prelude (C) *65*

  7.   *Coping with Communication Challenges: Answering*
      Your Most Pressing "Why" Questions about Speech (C) . . *69*

  8.   *Answering Your Most Pressing "Why" Questions*
      about Eating/Swallowing (C) *85*

  9.   *Answering Your Most Pressing "Why" Questions*
      about Walking/Mobility (C) *93*

  10. *Answering Your Most Pressing "Why" Questions*
      about Cognition/Memory (C) *107*

Table of Contents

11. Answering Your Most Pressing "Why" Questions
    about Social/Emotional Behaviors (C) 115

12. Dressing for Success (C&S) 121

13. HELP is not a Four- Letter Word: Learning How, Who,
    & When to Ask (C). 127

PART 2 What's Next? Homecoming 133

14. Prepare for Homecoming Before You
    Leave the Hospital (C). 135

15. A Caregiver's Guide to Sanity & Rewarding Rituals (C) 143

16. Back in the Game: Visitors & Community
    Reintegration (C&S). 147

17. Managing your Mindset & Finding Meaning (C&S) . . . 153

18. "Tapping" Down Anxiety, Pain, & Overwhelm (C&S). . 165

19. Getting on Autopilot (C&S). 175

20. The Simple Math Formula to Nutritional Wellness
    Through Food (C&S) 185

21. When To Rest: Balancing Fatigue against Pushing
    for Progress (C&S) 197

22. Let's Get Physical: Yep, I'm Talking Sex (C&S) 205

23. Powering Your Goals With "Why" Fuel (C&S) 217

PART 3 What Now?
       Making it Work When Everyone Leaves. 225

24. Restoring Routines (C&S). 227

25. Getting Your Life Back (C&S) 239

26. Driving & Working (C&S) 245

27. Some Days are Crappy (C&S) 255

28. Plowing through Plateaus (C&S) 261

29. Forgiveness, Acceptance, & Reinvention (C&S) 267

Parting Words 279

Appendix: Resources That Make Life Easier 281

Glossary of Types of Strokes 301

Glossary of Terms 305

Index 317

Bibliography 321

Suggested Readings 327

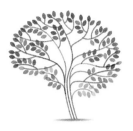

PREFACE

Why am I beginning this book on stroke recovery with the steps to recognize a stroke and respond quickly? Because the National Stroke Association tells us that at least one in four stroke survivors is at risk for having another stroke in their lifetime. In fact, within the first 5 years after a stroke occurs, the possibility of another stroke can increase by more than 40 percent.

Recognize a Stroke and Respond Quickly

Ask the person to:

SMILE: Check to see if one side of the face is drooping

RAISE ARMS: Notice weakness in arms or legs

SPEAK: Listen for slurred words or nonsense words

Call 911 immediately.

Seek rapid medical attention to preserve brain function.

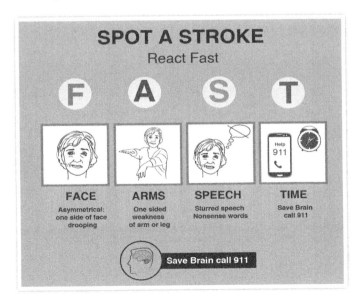

Additional symptoms that may signal a stroke

- Sudden difficulty seeing in one or both eyes.
- Severe dizziness and/or sudden loss of balance, coordination, or ability to walk.
- *Sudden* and severe headache for no reason. These headaches are called "thunderclap headaches," because of their suddenness and severity.

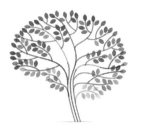

FOREWORD

In life, there are people who are deeply enlightened and are called to guide us. Like angels, they provide a light to illuminate our way. Tsgoyna Tanzman is one of these rare individuals. She has written this insightful guide that provides a light through the unknown and often dark maze that can overwhelm survivors and caregivers after a stroke. Her practical wisdom flows with answers, tools, and resources she gathered while she worked with stroke survivors for more than twenty-five years. Her experience as a speech-language pathologist, certified personal life coach, master practitioner of neuro-linguistic programming (NLP), and certified Mental Emotional Release Practitioner® come together to provide a perspective to the incredible healing power of hope.

I am grateful to her for sharing her knowledge and expertise with all those seeking help. She is a rare gem whose heartfelt hand of hope awaits you.

Blessings,

Valerie Greene

America's Stroke Coach
Founder & CEO Global Stroke Resource, Inc. aka Bcenter
Speaker, Author of *Conquering Stroke.*

INTRODUCTION

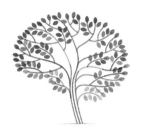

Hope is being able to see that there is light despite all of the darkness.
~ **Desmond Tutu** ~

Y ou are in the right place at the right time. You've chosen this book because you want answers, but who is it for? The caregiver? The stroke survivor? Family? Friends? *YES.*

Approximately 800,000 people a year in the United States have a stroke, but that's just a statistic.

Someone you love had a stroke.

I entered the darkened room to find my newly admitted "bleed" in Bed B.

Chase lay in his bed with a half-shaved head that revealed the stapled skull incision of a freshly repaired brain aneurysm. The other half of his head was a thick clump of stringy hair. Aesthetics are the last thing on anyone's mind when they've experienced a brain bleed.

I reached for the pair of glasses on his bedside table and extended them as I announced myself. "Hi, Chase, I'm Tsgoyna, your speech therapist." I watched for signs of comprehension and any ability to communicate, hoping he'd reach for his glasses and put them on. His entire right side lay paralyzed. He reached with his left hand and struggled to put the wire-rim glasses on his face. They were lopsided and smudged as if they'd been cleaned with butter. Chase opened his mouth and out came a torrent of incoherent gibberish, a flood of fractured syllables and sounds containing not one meaningful word. I

---

gently touched his hand and smiled, though my gut ached knowing the severity of his problem. He gripped my hand and his eyes widened in that pleading frightened way.

I squeezed back more firmly, saying, "It's going to be okay. Really, it is. I promise, we'll get you through this."

His face softened and his eyes looked more curious than scared.

"Are you in?" I asked.

He sighed, bowed his head, and then managed the tiniest, half-paralyzed smile as his eyes filled with hope.

This book is for and about the survivor's and their caregiver's recovery, and about the process of getting their lives back. Getting one's life back is a collaborative process, with different people taking the lead at different times. In the initial stages a caregiver leads. As recovery progresses, the survivor will increasingly participate. Family and friends will find the information and personal stories in these pages both hopeful and helpful in understanding the effects of a stroke, the intricacies of recovery, and how to be supportive as their loved one heals.

No one can predict how much a stroke will impact them in the short or long run but, most importantly, what you need now is hope, support, and answers.

"I just want my old life back," says every stroke survivor.

While there's no magic rewind button, *Hope After Stroke: The Holistic Guide to Getting Your Life Back,* gives you the information, tools, resources, and confidence you need to guide you along your journey.

Hope After Stroke is an evidence-based, holistic, practical, simple, and common-sense guide. While common sense isn't always common practice and simple doesn't always mean easy, this book offers you practical tips to make recovery possible and, dare I say, *hopeful.*

What exactly does *holistic* mean? Here "holistic" means looking at the *whole* person, taking into account the person's mind, body, spirit, and social factors, rather than just addressing the physical symptoms of a disease or injury.

Hope After Stroke is about recovering, discovering, and designing a new, productive, and meaningful life, whether there is total recovery or not.

The book is divided into three main sections that follow the course of recovery across major chunks of time:

Part 1: What Happened? *Life In the Hospital*

Part 2: What's Next? *Homecoming*

Part 3: What Now? *Making It Work When Everyone Leaves*

Chapters will include designations of "C" for Caregiver and/ or "S" for Survivor to help you find the sections written with you in mind. Refer to the Table of Contents for quick navigation.

At the end of every chapter is an **Essential Takeaway** that provides the most important information in bulleted form. You can skip right to the **Takeaways** for a quick overview of the chapter—a sort of "info to-go."

Essential Answers are also provided for each of the questions in Chapters 7 through 11 about Communication, Eating, Walking/ Mobility, Cognition/Memory, and Social/Emotional Behaviors.

In Part 1, caregivers will learn the working terminology of the type of stroke your Loved One (LO) experienced; why and how you have to be at the center of the rehab team; and what types of therapists will help with early recovery. I'll answer some of your most pressing "Why?" questions about Walking, Talking, Communication, Eating, Memory/Cognition, and Social/Emotional issues, and teach you how to reduce your risk of recurrent strokes. You'll learn how changing your language shapes your reality and why dressing for success jumpstarts recovery. You'll discover the "secret sauce" of exceptional recovering through the stories of *regular* people. Finally, you will learn why "help" is not a four-letter word but a necessary request, and why asking for it will be a gift to everyone.

In Part 2, you'll gain those "I'm glad somebody told me that" tips that make homecoming easier, *before* you leave the hospital. Caregivers will get their own guide to sanity. You'll learn how managing your mindset, finding meaning, and engaging in daily routines and rituals can speed up recovery and make success more likely. Survivors will learn practical strategies for dealing with visitors and reintegrating with their communities. Caregivers will discover the simple math formula for nutritional wellness; how to help your LO set goals, balance fatigue and rest; and how to "tap" down anxiety without medication. We'll talk about sex, and you'll get answers and resources for a touchy topic that is almost never discussed.

In Part 3, you'll learn to define what getting your life back really means as well as how to make *life* your therapy. You'll gain knowledge about working and driving and how to plow through apparent recovery plateaus. You'll learn the science behind how forgiveness alters one's brain and how acceptance and reinvention are possible. Finally, you'll get a hefty selection of resources and product recommendations that make life easier, facilitate recovery, and preserve everyone's dignity.

As a speech-language pathologist, master practitioner of neuro-linguistic programming (NLP), and a life coach for over 25 years, I've journeyed with thousands of stroke survivors and their families through every phase of recovery from hospitalization to coming home, to returning to work, and even up to 20 years after a person's stroke. I've worked with survivors in hospitals, residential settings, clinics, home care, and community settings. I've witnessed "miracles," where people have reached levels of growth that defied the grimmest predictions and prognoses.

I know therapy is hard work, but when mixed with a reframed perspective, humor, appreciation, and gratitude, recovery can also be exciting and *transformative*.

What's the most important thing my families have said helped them recover?

HOPE

That's what I am offering you. Hope, answers, and practical tools.

I'm offering you the knowledge and the hope you can do this. The promise you can have both a reason and a desire to get up in the morning. The promise you and your loved one can recover and have a life worth living.

This is *your* journey. I'm only a guide. You are the Explorer and soon-to-be Expert.

Know I'm here with you and for you.

Yes, you can get through this.

Yes, you will get through this.

Yes, you must get through this.

Take a breath. Close your eyes and tell yourself aloud…

"Yes, I can."

"Yes, I must."

"Yes, I will."

Every journey, no matter how long, begins with a single step. So, let's begin yours, now.

PART 1
What Happened?
Life in the Hospital

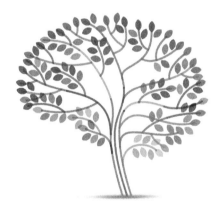

WHAT'S IN A NAME? GET TO KNOW YOUR STROKE (C)

It is much more important to know what sort of a patient has a disease than what sort of a disease a patient has.
~ William Osler ~
A founding professor of Johns Hopkins Hospital

Someone in the U.S. has a stroke about once every 40 seconds.

WHAT REALLY HAPPENS?

A stroke is an *event* where the brain is deprived of oxygen, either by a blockage or a bleed causing destruction of brain tissue. Strokes may occur in many parts of the brain so they're also described by their location. Depending on where the stroke occurs different neurological outcomes may appear. (See the glossary for a listing of the types of strokes.)

Essentially strokes fall into two different categories:

Blocks and Bleeds

BLOCK: *An ischemic (is-KEY-mick) stroke*

What happens?

Most strokes are caused by a blockage, which can be one of two types. When a clot or plaque inside a blood vessel blocks oxygen and nutrients from getting to the body's cells, this is called a *thrombosis*. If a blood clot originates in another area of the body, such as the heart, and travels to the brain causing vessel blockage, it's called an *embolism.*

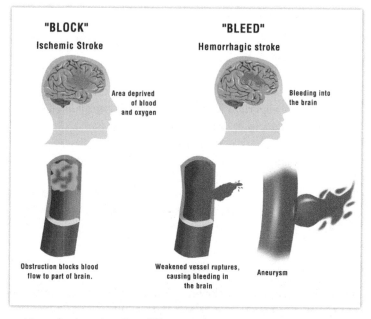

Vessels showing the difference between obstruction and weakened states

BLEED: A hemorrhagic (HEM-or-rah-jic) stroke

What happens?

During a hemorrhagic stroke, a blood vessel leaks or bursts, resulting in bleeding inside the brain. This causes cells to die because their supply of glucose and oxygen is interrupted. Causes of hemorrhagic stroke can include high blood pressure; aneurysm (AN-your-ism), which is a weakening in the wall of a blood vessel; or an arteriovenous (are-TEAR-ee-o-VEEN-us) malformation (AVM), which is a group of abnormally tangled blood vessels. Aneurysms and AVMs are often called the brain's ticking time bombs because these abnormalities may be present at birth, but will have no symptoms until they burst.

Hemorrhagic strokes are less common than blockages by 20%, but they account for more than 30% of all stroke deaths. There are two types of hemorrhages: intracerebral and subarachnoid hemorrhages, which are differentiated by their location and cause. See the chart below to learn more

TWO TYPES OF HEMORRHAGIC STROKE		
Type	Location	Cause
Intracerebral	Bleeding **within** the brain	High blood pressure. Burst aneurysm within the brain.
Subarachnoid	The area between the brain and the skull. It is filled with cerebrospinal fluid (CSF), which acts as a floating cushion to protect the brain.	An artery on or near the surface of brain bursts. May be genetic and present at birth. Falls or other head trauma.

Swelling is an additional danger of a brain bleed

Swelling, also known as *intracranial pressure* (ICP), or edema, causes the brain to push against the hard, inflexible skull (or cranium). The counter-compression of the skull pushing against the brain, further reduces the brain's blood supply and oxygen. Brain swelling is so serious that, if left uncontrolled and elevated, it may lead to death. To relieve ICP, an accurate diagnosis and prompt medical or surgical treatment is crucial.

In addition to blocks and bleeds, there are also mini-strokes.

MINI-STROKE: TRANSIENT ISCHEMIC ATTACK (TIA)
What happens?

A mini-stroke, or *transient ischemic attack* (TIA) resembles a full-blown stroke except for two major differences. A TIA is brief and fleeting and the blockage of blood flow to the brain is temporary, or *transient* in time. Typically there is no tissue death or permanent damage from a TIA. These symptoms appear and last less than 24 hours before disappearing.

However, don't let the unassuming name fool you. *A TIA is a huge warning sign.* Statistics show that forty percent of those who have a TIA will later have an actual stroke with nearly half those strokes occurring within the next few days. *Seek medical attention immediately to address the underlying problems.*

What's happening to the brain during the "acute" phase of the stroke?

Within minutes of an artery being blocked during an ischemic stroke, two different zones of damage occur. The first zone of damage closest to the blocked artery is known as the *core* and it is the spot where nerve cells (*neurons*) die because of a lack of oxygen and glucose (the cell's vital nutrients). While these neurons in the core unfortunately cannot be revived, they are surrounded by an even larger area called the *penumbra.* *The penumbra* is the secondary zone of damage. Think of the penumbra surrounding the core like the concentric circle around a bull's-eye. The neurons in the penumbra are fragile and barely alive; first, because they're still not getting their full supply of blood and oxygen and second, because swelling in the area causes a toxic mix of chemicals that interferes with nerve function. However, the penumbra has the potential for recovery.

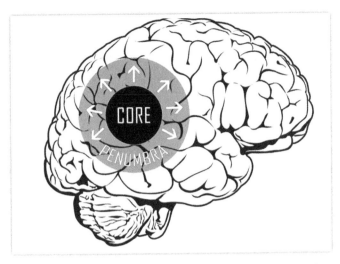

The core is the area of dead neurons. The penumbra has billions of stunned neurons that can recover.

What do I mean by this? Well, imagine your brain is a freeway system with many roads branching to other superhighways and connector roads. Now, picture a tornado damaging a major portion of the freeway. At the *core* of the destruction, the road is obliterated. Aside from the core destruction, there is debris and damage obstructing some of the connector roads, making them temporarily impassable. These roads are not functional, but they're intact enough to make them eventually reparable. In the brain, this area is the *penumbra*.

So, how is the penumbra the area of recovery?

As stated above, the neurons in the penumbra are alive, but in a state of shock. In other words, there is damage at the core, but the surrounding area is salvageable. But time is of the essence because these neurons in the penumbra region can still die off if blood flow isn't reestablished quickly. One of the goals of treatment is to break up the clot and get blood back into the ischemic area. Medications like tPA, known as the clot-busting drug, allow blood flow to be reestablished, but only if administered within the first three to four hours of the onset of stroke symptoms. These precious but vulnerable nerve cells in the penumbra hold the *potential* for recovery *if* they are activated. So, what's the "magic wand" that wakes them up and recruits them into action? Physical and mental activity.

Not so fast, though. In this *acute phase of recovery*, which is defined as the first seven days after the onset of stroke symptoms, the brain is in a vulnerable position. **Too much physical or mental stimulation too soon will have a negative effect on recovery.** That's why limiting visitors, optimizing a calm environment, and minimizing external stressors, are essential. See Chapter 2: Advocating for Your Loved One for strategies to manage recovery during this phase.

Although your loved one (LO) is not a newborn, approaching them with the same energy of security, calm, love, and tenderness, is an important part of relating to the frightened and vulnerable person during this phase. A calm environment promotes self-healing because the body's stress response is not activated by its surroundings.

For the acute phase, think *less is more*. Short periods of small amounts of stimulation are adequate. In fact, it's absolutely essential to *not* do too much too soon.

During this acute phase, a doctor may order physical, occupational, and speech therapists to perform evaluations and assess your LO's safety, mobility, and cognitive function. Physical therapists may passively range your LO's limbs to help maintain muscle length and preserve healthy joint movement before initiating active therapy. Occupational therapists may assess vision, sensory skills, range of movement (ROM) of arms and hands, and bathroom abilities. Speech therapists will evaluate eating and communication skills. In Chapter 3, we'll discuss your rehab team in depth: who they are, what they do, and why you yourself are a critical member of the team.

In his book *Stronger After Stroke*, Peter G. Levine, gives us a simple way to identify the phases of recovery by means of a timeline.

He encourages us to know the timeline in order to take advantage of each phase.

Levine's Stroke Recovery Timeline

Hyperacute Phase: *The first six hours from the onset of symptoms.*

Acute Phase: *The first seven days after the onset of symptoms.*

Subacute Phase: *The first seven days to three months after the onset of symptoms.* This is known as the "sweet spot" of recovery because during this phase the most rapid progress can be made.

Chronic Phase: *Three months after stroke, continuing for the rest of the survivor's life.*

Connections are Everything

Ideally, active therapy should begin when your LO shows signs of moving into the subacute phase; however, because of shorter hospital stays, sometimes intervention begins while a person is still in the acute stage of recovery. What are the signs someone is moving into the subacute phase of recovery?

First, things will begin to improve without any effort. This is called *spontaneous recovery.* You might notice tiny finger movements where previously there were none. A foot may wiggle. Speech may show some improvement. This is where a caregiver's observations are vital to the team because you likely spend more time with the survivor and will notice subtle or large improvements that therapists may miss. These readiness signs mean neurons in the penumbra are coming "online" again and are primed for active engagement. This is a window of opportunity for stimulating neurons. This is done by challenging them to connect and form new neural pathways.

How do we challenge the survivor? Stimulation and therapy. Why does this help? It helps because we are harnessing the growth potential of *neuroplasticity.*

Neuroplasticity is the brain's spectacular ability to change and reorganize itself by growing new neural pathways and synaptic connections. "Neuro" is a prefix that means "neuron." "Plastic" here doesn't mean the material, but instead means that those neurons are changeable, malleable, and modifiable.

This relatively new discovery from the early 1970s means there is more hope than ever for stroke recovery. Neuroplasticity is all about connections. Check out the math: there are approximately 100 billion nerve cells in the brain and an estimated quadrillion (1000 trillion) connections between neurons. Considering that a typical stroke kills less than two billion neurons (only 2% of total brain cells) that leaves a lot of viable and malleable material for the survivor and their team to work with! It turns out the number of *connections* between living neurons matters more than the number of isolated dead or alive neurons. In short, the number of living neurons awaiting connection is more important to stroke recovery than the number of dead neurons.

How do we rewire the recovering neurons in the penumbra? Rewiring the brain means creating new connections by getting working neurons to wire together. Repetitive thoughts, activities, and behaviors change the brain's structure and function. For better or worse, neuroplasticity shapes every brain, even undamaged ones.

According to Dr. Norman Doidge, psychiatrist and researcher at Columbia University, as well as the author of *The Brain that Changes Itself,* "[Neuroplasticity] renders our brains not only more resourceful but also more vulnerable to outside influences. Neuroplasticity has the power to produce more flexible but also more rigid behaviors. Ironically some of our most stubborn habits and disorders are products of our plasticity. Once a particular plastic change occurs in the brain and becomes well established, it can prevent other changes from occurring."

If our brains build connections by the thoughts we think and the behaviors and activities we choose to perform, then we better be vigilant about what we're thinking and doing. In Chapter 17, you'll learn more about how managing your mindset is critical for both the caregiver and survivor in the recovery process. Persistent worry and negative "stinkin' thinkin'" will only lead to the development of a fast-track anxious neural network that makes faith, hope, and optimism harder to achieve.

If you want a more positive future, you have to practice a more positive present. You must focus on beliefs that state the body and brain are resilient and restorative. Use a magnifying-glass approach to look for evidence of improvement and what's working. Whatever you magnify will continue to be magnified. Whatever you appreciate, to use a financial term, appreciates, so *appreciate* small improvements. It's just as easy to build a good habit as it is to establish a bad one. It's all in what you repeatedly think and do. In Chapter 19: Getting on Autopilot, you'll learn how and why implementing repetitive routines develops stronger neural connections and conserves brain energy.

Whether it's relearning how to open and close a hand, tie a shoe, play an instrument, or maintain a positive mental attitude, the brain learns through repetitive practice.

This is the basis of recovery.

Wow, that was a long way of saying:

> *Just do it. Do it again. Then, do it again.*
> *Be vigilant. Make sure the things you're doing and repeating are the things you want.*

ESSENTIAL TAKEAWAYS

- A stroke is a loss of blood and oxygen (caused by either by a blockage or a bleed) that destroys brain tissue.
- The *core* is the site of dead brain cells caused by the stroke.
- The *penumbra* surrounds the core and is the site of stunned but alive neurons (or nerve cells.). Recovery depends on reestablishing the blood supply, oxygen, and glucose to these neurons as well as recruiting them to connect through repetitive activity at the right time in the recovery process.

- The number of connector neurons is far greater and more important to recovery than the total number of dead or alive neurons in the brain.

- *Neuroplasticity* is the brain's ability to change, grow, reorganize, and rewire itself.

- The Four Phases of Recovery, moving forward through time: Hyperacute, Acute, Subacute, and Chronic.

- In the Acute Phase (from the sixth hour to seven days after a stroke), the brain is in a delicate stage. The caregiver should focus on keeping the survivor calm and safe. Limit stimulation and visitors. Follow passive range of motion exercises. Look for spontaneous recovery (or improvement with no effort) as it signals the start of the subacute phase.

- The Subacute Phase (the period from seven days to approximately three months after the onset of stroke) is the most important phase for recovery because neurons are coming alive. Stimulation, therapy, and neuroplasticity at this phase lead to the highest level of recovery.

- Repetition of behavior grows new neural pathways. Recovery depends on vast repetitions of behavior.

ADVOCATING FOR YOUR LOVED ONE (C)

If you're going through hell, keep going.
~ Winston Churchill ~

WHY A CAREGIVER IS NEEDED

I'm a firm believer that it is easier to prevent a problem than to solve one. With that in mind, I want to share some facts with you. These may be disturbing, but please know that they are mentioned to reinforce the idea that a caregiver is dearly needed at the hospital when a loved one is in the early stages of recovery.

The statistics about U.S. hospital medical errors, including those taking place at good hospitals, are alarming. At last count it was the equivalent of a Boeing 747 crashing everyday with all of the people aboard killed. I don't say this to bash hospital staff or to terrify you, but to illuminate the truth and the *necessity* for someone advocating for your loved one.

I've witnessed food delivered to a highly allergic patient who could not talk or advocate for herself. Three signs posted in highly visible locations read:

> PATIENT ALLERGIC:
> NO FLOWERS, CHEESE, OR EGGS.

Yet, her breakfast tray arrived with a cheese omelet and a carnation.

I averted another crisis when a patient *nearly* received the wrong gastric tube feeding because of a mix-up in patients' names. Luckily

I read the name on the bag and stopped the aide before anything went wrong.

There is no beating around the bush. Someone needs to be with your LO during their first few days of hospitalization, *or longer,* because the survivor needs to feel safe. It's not that hospitals aren't safe, but your LO is in a very compromised physical and mental state and will likely be terrified when they become aware of what's happened.

Fear inhibits healing. Safety allows the nervous system to relax. Even in the absence of apparent consciousness, creating a tone of security and love is critical. Several survivors have shared with me that they remember hearing the staff talking about them— everything from snide remarks about them being fat to admonitions to their caregivers about their unlikely recovery and poor prognosis.

You, or another trusted person, can observe, question, and follow up with the nurses, doctors, and rehab team to make sure your LO receives the most appropriate and best care as their condition changes. Even under the best circumstances, information gets lost, miscommunicated, and misinterpreted.

First and foremost, a caregiver is needed because your LO trusts you and knows you understand them. For instance, you know if they wear a hearing aid, glasses, or contact lenses to function normally. Be certain to tell the doctor and nurses if your LO wears contact lenses. This is an often-overlooked detail that can cause significant irreparable visual damage if contact lenses are left in a person's eyes.

Your LO will likely also need help doing or getting things to aid in their comfort and immediate needs, and they may not be able to speak or use a call button to summon help. You may need to assist your LO in ordering and eating food, using the bathroom, and getting dressed.

Second, a caregiver is needed because your presence signals a sense of certainty and security to the survivor. Something as simple as changing rooms or beds can be very disorienting and alarming to your LO.

Third, because you are likely to spend more time with your LO than anyone else, you'll be the first to see signs of trouble or progress. Reporting changes to your nurse is crucial to your LO's wellbeing; it also allows you to make decisions about urgent, of-the-moment matters.

Fourth, a caregiver is needed to truly advocate for their loved one's recovery and treatment. Hospitals are in the *business* of healing people. Like any business, they must take in more money than they spend. They get this money from insurance companies, and as we know, it's not always easy to get insurance companies to pay up. Generally, the criteria for an insurance company to pay for and authorize more treatment is a patient's progress. *Progress justifies payment.* Where it gets murky is knowing exactly what that criteria for progress entails. Every insurance company is different, and as therapy progresses, their criteria may change.

Your LO will have a case manager (CM) who is the liaison between the hospital and the insurance company. The case manager will also assist with discharge planning. See Chapter 14: Prepare for Homecoming Before You Leave the Hospital. Your job as caregiver is to create an alliance with your CM and **help them understand who your LO is as a real person connected to a real life, not just another case number with a bottom line.** Ask the CM specific questions about the insurance company's requirements to continue authorizing treatment. Be sincere and appreciative of their help and alliance.

There's a point where being an *advocate* may be perceived as being a demanding pain, but you must be persistent. Once you know what criteria your LO needs to meet in order to qualify for services, you must *make sure* they receive those services regularly. If a therapy session is cancelled because your LO was sleeping, ask your therapy team to reschedule it.

In addition, make sure *any and all progress your LO makes is documented in the medical charts.* Progress doesn't always happen in a therapy session, so *if you see something, say something.* Make sure it's recorded by either the nurses or the therapists. **You always have the right to see your medical records.**

Fifth and finally, a caregiver is needed because while your LO is the most important person to you, they are *one of many* most important people on a recovery ward. Nursing staff is often short (with ratios of 1 nurse to 10 patients), and attending to everyone as quickly as one hopes is just not possible.

WHY A CAREGIVER NEEDS *SELF-CARE*

You can't do and be all. It's a known fact in the medical community that a solitary caregiver runs a tremendous risk for burnout, illness, and/or depression.

You must recognize and honor your needs for food, rest, and self-care. Ask for help. Arrange break times with another friend or family member. Bring supplies to aid in your comfort for long days at the hospital. Here's a short list of hospital essentials to make caregivers more comfortable:

- A warm, soft sweater or jacket, a light blanket, and a pillow
- A cell phone, cord, charger, and backup battery
- A computer with charger
- Headphones
- Healthy snacks
- A water bottle

Allowing a friend or family member to give you even a short break, like a shower, or a nap in your own bed, will revive you. You may not have to be at your LO's bedside 24 hours a day, depending on their level of alertness and communication, but you may. If you choose to stay overnight, ask if the hospital can provide some reasonable accommodation such as a reclining chair or even an additional bed. You will need your energy and mental sharpness in the coming weeks, so taking care of yourself from the get-go is crucial.

When are the most important times to be with your loved one?

You won't always know in advance when the following activities will occur, but it's a good idea to regularly check-in with the nursing staff to find out if any of these are planned. Do your best to be with your loved one during:

- *Transfers:* When he or she is moved to a different bed or ward. It is very disorienting to be moved to a new location and can be physically, cognitively, and emotionally stressing.

- *Medical Procedures:* MRI, CT scans, videofluoroscopy, ultrasounds, blood draws, heparin injections, etc., may need to be performed, and your LO will feel safer if you're there to go through it with them.

- *Meal Times:* This includes gastric tube feedings, during which you can assist with eating and monitoring for signs of difficulty.

Hospital Tip: Assume the best, but remain vigilant. If something is not right, speak up.

Here are a few situations when you may need to speak up:

- If you ever observe questionable safety violations, you must speak up. Are caregivers observing standard hygiene procedures, like handwashing and using gloves?

- Are staff checking the survivor's hospital wristband before any procedure, food, or medication is performed or given? In order to reduce human error, most hospitals use wristband scanners to confirm a person's identity.

- Are staff placing the call button on your LO's functional side, so they can call for assistance getting to the bathroom? (More falls occur because patients attempt to go to the bathroom by themselves when no help comes).

Who to Talk To

Begin with the head nurse. Establish a respectful and appreciative tone and objectively state the problem, but most importantly, state what *solution or outcome* you want instead. Most people focus exclusively on the problem. By requesting the outcome or solution you want in the most positive way, you create a higher likelihood that it will be done.

What Can Go Wrong during Hospitalization?

Regrettably and potentially a lot—infections, medical complications from other preexisting conditions, intolerance to new medications, agitation, and delirium. Prolonged bed rest increases a patient's possibility for skin ulcers and breakdown, as well as the formation of blood clots in leg veins. Swallowing disorders increase the chance of bacteria entering the patient's lungs and causing pneumonia. (See Chapter 8: Answering Your Most Pressing "Why" Questions about Eating/Swallowing). In addition, any time there is a presence of tubes in either the lungs, stomach, or bladder, bacteria can migrate past the skin and cause internal infections.

During the acute phase of stroke recovery, about 25% of stroke survivors may experience delirium or a condition called *ICU psychosis*. For the survivor, it's an acute, transient, and fluctuating disorder of consciousness, attention, and cognition resulting in delirium. For the caregiver, it's very scary and confusing. About one out of every three patients who spends more than five days in an intensive care unit (ICU) experiences some form of psychotic reaction.

Don't Expect It, but Recognize It— What Does ICU Psychosis Look Like?

Your loved one may be experiencing ICU psychosis if they become agitated, severely anxious, restless, hallucinatory, disoriented, paranoid, delusional, and/or exhibit fluctuating levels of consciousness from passive to aggressive to combative.

ICU psychosis can be caused by both environmental and medical factors

Environmental Factors Leading to ICU Psychosis:

- **Sensory Overload:** Hospitals are noisy places with machines beeping, carts moving, and unfamiliar people entering and exiting rooms at all hours. Numerous people may ask your LO questions and give them instructions, often in ways that are too fast and incomprehensible for a person in the hyperacute and acute stages of a new stroke to comprehend and obey.

- **Stress:** Patients are anxious and fearful and may not be able to speak or comprehend what is happening. As a result, they may feel helpless to control their situation. I've often heard a person recall, "I remember everyone talking and yelling around me and I was trying to talk, but people didn't listen, didn't answer me, didn't respond. I didn't know what was happening."

- **Sensory Deprivation:** A survivor in the ICU may be isolated from family, friends, and familiar, comfortable surroundings. What's more, they may not have access to eyeglasses or hearing aids.

- **Sleep Deprivation and Disturbance:** Hospital staff routinely interrupt patients' sleep to draw blood, administer medication, and check vitals.

- **Continuous, Unnatural Light Levels:** An absence of windows and natural light may disrupt the normal biorhythms of day and night orientation.

- **Lack of Orientation:** A survivor can lose awareness of time, date, and place, especially if they're moved to a different room.

Medical Factors Leading to ICU Psychosis:

- **Dehydration**
- **Pain**
- **Metabolic Disturbances:** These may include an electrolyte imbalance, *hypoxia* (low blood oxygen levels), or elevated liver enzymes.
- **Medication Side Effects:** These may be related to the administration of new drugs never before taken. Alternatively, if your LO routinely took a medication but it was not reported in the medical history, negative side

effects may occur. For instance, missing even a single dose of an antidepressant such as Effexor® can result in severe head buzzing and delirium.

- **Infection:** Infections create fever and toxins in the body, even in cases as basic as urinary tract infections or contact lenses that haven't been removed.

How is ICU Psychosis Managed?

Finding the cause or source of the disturbance results in the best treatment.

To do this, the nursing staff and doctors will:

- Perform a thorough review of medications, levels of hydration and vitals, and treat any infections.
- Possibly administer haloperidol or another medication for psychosis (antipsychotics), especially if a person is attempting to remove IVs or other monitoring devices.
- Possibly use restraints if a person is trying to exit the bed or room and presents a danger to himself.

Here's a list of things you can do to help the nursing staff and doctors identify ICU psychosis and reduce its incidence in the first place:

- Notify nursing and medical staff of concerns (including smelly urine, as it may be a sign of a urinary tract infection).
- Limit sensory stimulation in your LO's room to protect their sleep.
- Reduce extraneous noise and interruptions.
- Limit the number of visitors and keep visits brief. Do not allow sick friends to visit!
- If the hospital *allows,* use lavender essential oil, which is known for its calming effects. Put drops on your LO's pillow and hospital gown, or provide a diffuser that disperses essential oil into the air. (Again, check for the safety compliance of using a diffuser in a hospital room, especially in the ICU.)

- Make sure your LO has access to their eyeglasses or hearing aids, if previously used.

What Can Go Right during Hospitalization?

In a perfect scenario, a stroke survivor wakes up, recognizes others, is oriented, and comprehends things. They may progress quickly through self-care skills like using the bathroom, eating and drinking, and dressing themselves with minimal problems. Their physical abilities may rapidly improve in regards to standing, balancing, and walking. Speech may show rapid signs of recovery. The nursing staff may communicate well with the survivor and family and progress is seen daily.

Tips for Thanking Nurses

Nurses, doctors, and support staff commit their lives to serving the most ill and needy in our society. Most are called to this work because of their true compassion and a strong belief in helping people heal. They are tireless givers and they often do it at a huge personal expense. They may work ridiculously long shifts of 12- to 14-hour days under relentless demands and high stress from patients, families, and supervising hospital staff. We *expect* care providers to be perfect, and to attend to our needs as if we were the only ones they were serving, but they are human. Humans sometimes make mistakes or simply aren't at their peak level of performance. The best way to make sure your LO is safe is by being present and getting to know and *appreciate* the nursing staff, until your LO is capable of advocating for himself.

Show your nurses the gratitude and appreciation they deserve. Know their names, smile, and say thank you often. A sincere personal note of thanks and recognition means more than you know. Send a praise letter to their supervisors. Bring small gifts of healthy foods, good coffee, or other treats.

ESSENTIAL TAKEAWAYS

- You, a trusted family member, or friend need to be with your Loved One as consistently as possible during their first week of hospitalization.

- You are the advocate and voice for your LO who can't speak or properly care for themselves.

- Caregivers need breaks. ASK FOR HELP. Bring essential comforts for your long days at the hospital: a sweater, cell phone and charger, computer and charger, headphones, healthy snacks, and a refillable water bottle.

- If you see something, say something. Report a patient's progress or problems to the nursing staff.

- Report unusual behaviors or concerns to nursing staff, including smelly urine as it may be a sign of a urinary tract infection (UTI).

- Know your nurses' names, smile, and say thank you often. Write a sincere personal note of thanks, or send a praise letter to nursing supervisors. Bring small treats for nurses to show you care.

YOU ARE THE CENTER OF YOUR REHAB TEAM (C&S)

We join spokes together in a wheel, but it is the center hole that makes the wagon move.

~ Lao Tzu ~

FOCUS ON THE PROGRESS, *NOT* THE PROGNOSIS

Surviving a stroke is the first stage of recovery.

How much recovery one will need and how long it will take are your most urgent questions, but regrettably, there are no *definitive* answers because each person and each injury can be so different. But that can be good news. While obvious signs of rapid improvement are encouraging, even initially severe impairments may radically shift during the subsequent stages of recovery.

One of the most difficult challenges for stroke survivors and their families is the uncertainty of what will happen next. For that reason I encourage caregivers to look for signs of a loved one's *progress* rather than focus on the potential limitations of their *prognosis*. This is one reason why YOU are the most important part of the rehab team. That means both You, the Survivor, and You, the Caregiver. In the initial stages the caregiver will be more involved, but as recovery continues, the survivor will increasingly take the lead and take responsibility for their own progress.

HOW AND WHY THE *SURVIVOR* IS INTEGRAL TO THE REHAB TEAM

Why? The simple answer is that no one cares more about your life than you do. Your input is essential to help your team assist you in meeting your emotional and physical needs, determining your strengths and limitations, and supporting you in achieving your goals and recovering a life that's productive and meaningful.

In the earliest days and weeks of your recovery, you will depend upon others for assistance, and you will do your best to follow your doctors' and therapists' instructions, but it's important that you become an *active* team member, not just a passive recipient of services. You and your team will work together to achieve your highest level of independence.

HOW AND WHY THE *CAREGIVER* IS INTEGRAL TO THE REHAB TEAM

You will be with your loved one many more hours a day than any other member of the rehab team. Therefore you will have a front-row seat to any signs of *spontaneous recovery.*

Spontaneous recovery is simply evidence of what the body does best—works to repair itself. What will it look like? *It will look like your LO is "getting better."* As the post-stroke brain recovers, shocked neurons in the penumbra wake up and are primed for communication with other neurons. This early stage of recovery is a critical period, because, if you recall, it is the *connections* between neurons that build new pathways.

Your LO's spontaneous improvement may be evident in some, or all, of the areas affected by the stroke, including sensation, balance, motor function, swallowing, understanding language, and speaking. The first three months following a stroke are when we typically see the fastest and greatest amount of recovery. It is crucial to remember that spontaneous recovery is just the start. Doctors often tell families at the end of three to six months that whatever your LO's level of improvement is at that point is "as good as it gets," but there are thousands of stroke survivors that disprove that every day. It's true that once the period of spontaneous recovery is past, progress will be slower and not so dramatic. The months that follow require more focused effort for the survivor to gain improvement, but as long as the brain is stimulated and used, survivors will continue to make progress.

Considering hospital therapy sessions range from 30 minutes to up to 3 or 4 hours a day, progress may not always take place under the supervision of a doctor or therapist. Instead, it's important that caregivers look for and report any signs of improvement in the areas of communication, eating, physical mobility, and social and emotional functioning. For communication, look for improvements in either understanding speech (receptive comprehension) and/ or speaking (expressive speech). Watch for improvements or problems with eating, chewing, or swallowing. Be alert to changes in physical mobility, as your LO may show improvement in either motor function or sensation in the fingers, hands, arms, elbows, and shoulders. Rolling over in bed or sitting up unassisted are evidence of motor-function progress. Look for movement and/ or improvement of sensation in the toes, ankles, knees, and legs. Finally, look for signs of improvement or difficulties in emotional status, and be sure to report these changes to the nursing staff, doctors, and any therapists who are treating your LO.

THE CAREGIVER BRIDGES THE GAP UNTIL THE SURVIVOR TAKES THE LEAD

If your LO has lost the ability to communicate either because of language impairments, memory and/or cognitive disturbances, you as the caregiver can help the rehab team by being the mouthpiece and advocate for your loved one. You have the big picture and broad perspective of who your LO is and was before the stroke. It's important your team learns and understands what they liked and disliked and *who they were and are* in order to help generate meaningful goals.

CONNECTIONS ARE EVERYTHING

Your connection with your rehab team mimics what the brain is striving to do for the stroke survivor—*connect.* Remember, *connections are everything.* Neurons that fire together wire together. A rehab team working together promotes the best outcome.

Since you've already mastered the medical terminology of stroke, learning a few more initials and "hospital speak" will be easy. So, besides doctors and nurses, let's get to know *who else* is on your team.

WHO IS ON YOUR REHAB TEAM?
WHAT DO THEY DO?

It might be helpful to think of your rehab team like a pit crew at a NASCAR race. In other words, they are a group of highly trained individuals with expertise in specialized areas working toward the common goal of getting the survivor on the road and back in the race. Rehabilitation teams and individualized treatment plans are specifically designed for each survivor based on their injury and needs, the facility's resources, and the survivor's insurance coverage. Typically the team is led by a *Physiatrist.*

- **Physiatrist** (FIZZ-eye-uh-trist): A special rehab medical doctor who's versed in the latest stroke recovery treatments. The physiatrist is the gatekeeper of the rehab team. They are responsible for ordering tests and directing services including all therapists and other specialists throughout the rehab process.

PLEASE NOTE:
A physiatrist is **NOT** *a psychiatrist, a doctor treating mental health,* **NOR** *a podiatrist, a doctor treating feet.*

Other members of the rehab team include:
- Occupational Therapist (OT)
- Physical Therapist (PT)
- Speech Therapist (ST)
- Social Worker: (SW)

It's common to have a core team of three therapists assessing your LO's current level of function: the occupational therapist (OT), physical therapist (PT), and speech therapist (ST). Although therapists realize your LO is a whole person, for practical purposes these three specialties divide the body into three parts.

OCCUPATIONAL THERAPY (OT)

What They Do: Retrain/enable survivors to use the bathroom, shower, dress, and eat

> *Body Systems Involved:*
> *From the neck to the trunk, including the arms and hands*

An occupational therapist's services may include:

- Assistance in recovery of Activities of Daily Living (ADLs) starting with bathroom hygiene. OTs focus on grooming, such as toothbrushing, face-washing, shaving, putting on makeup, hair-drying, toileting, showering and dressing.
- Body mechanics and strengthening for optimal balance and performance during ADLs.
- Retraining shoulder mobility and strength. Splinting limbs and providing slings.
- Retraining hand movements for grasping, writing and eating.
- Stabilizing tremulous hands.
- Sensory re-education/stimulation and tone management of a *spastic* (with too high, nearly rigid muscle tone) or *flaccid* (with too low, weak muscle tone) upper limbs.
- Visual retraining to reduce the impact of visual-field deficits and double vision, which can cause safety issues especially as related to mobility and neglect of the paralyzed side of the body.

- Perceptual retraining related to awareness of the survivor's body and environment.
- Cognitive re-education to facilitate the survivor's ability to plan and follow a daily routine using memory strategies, problem-solving skills, and organization.
- Environmental evaluations, recommendations, and modifications focusing on safety hazards and equipment used in the home.
- Caregiver training for safety, home exercise programs, and ADLs.

OTs may also diagnose and treat swallowing and feeding disorders. For instance, they may train the survivor on the mechanical aspect of feeding themselves by using constraint-induced therapy (CIT) to recover abilities in the affected paralyzed hand or provide compensatory strategies and tools for using the non-dominant hand.

PHYSICAL THERAPY (PT)
What They Do: Get survivors moving

> *Body Systems Involved:*
> *From the trunk down to the toes*

A physical therapist's services may include:

- Teaching bed mobility so that your LO can help position themselves in bed to sit up.
- Training for transfers including: from the bed to a chair to the bathroom, and ultimately to the car to go home.
- Sensory re-education/stimulation and tone management of a spastic (with too high, nearly rigid muscle tone) or flaccid (with too low, weak muscle tone) lower limb. (See Chapter 9: Answering Your Most Pressing "Why" Questions about Walking/Mobility.)

- Retraining mobility for walking or using the least restrictive device possible (e.g., wheelchairs, walkers, canes) to aid in mobility.
- Fitting patients with orthotic braces to stabilize ankles and feet for improved walking.
- Retraining the survivor in balance.
- Teaching Fall Recovery: how to get off the floor safely after a fall.

SPEECH THERAPY (ST)

What They Do: Get survivors communicating

Body Systems Involved:
From the neck up to the top of the head

Speech therapists may also be known as Speech-Language Pathologists (SLP). A speech pathologist's services may include:

- Diagnosing and assisting with feeding/swallowing issues also known as *dysphagia* (DIS-fay-zhuh). For more detailed information, see Chapter 8: Answering Your Most Pressing "Why" Questions about Eating/ Swallowing.
- Retraining speech communication due to *aphasia* (AH-fay-zhuh), or a loss of language. See Chapter 7: Coping With Communication Challenges for a full description of aphasia.
- Diagnosing and treating vocal disorders including breathy, whispered speech, paralyzed vocal cords, and vocal cords damaged from tracheostomy tubes and long-term intubation.
- Diagnosing and treating *dysarthria* (DIS-are-three-uh) (slow, uncoordinated speech due to weak muscles) or *apraxia* (Ah-PRAX-ee-uh) (motor planning problems with adequate muscle strength).

- Restoring cognitive functions such as short- and long-term memory, organization, planning, sequencing, and path-finding.
- Developing alternative communication systems if verbal speech is impossible.

BUT WAIT, THERE'S MORE... WHO *ELSE* MAY BE ON YOUR TEAM?

A stroke affects more than just the physical body and depending on your needs you may have other professionals help you address the emotional, psychological, logistical, and bureaucratic issues of recovery. These may include:

Social Workers (SW): Social workers help survivors manage insurance claims, file for disability, provide counseling, assist with social and emotional recovery, engage in vocational exploration, and obtain related services such as transportation and information regarding Power of Attorney and Advance Directives. See Chapter 11: Answering Your Most Pressing "Why" Questions about Social/Emotional Behaviors.

Psychiatrist, Psychologist, or Neuropsychologist: A healthcare provider or counselor who conducts cognitive tests to assess the survivor's thinking and learning abilities. They also help the survivor and their family adjust emotionally to life after stroke.

Case Managers (CM): Case managers act as the liaison between the hospital, the insurance company, and survivor. Make them your ally as they are crucial for getting insurance companies to authorize therapies. (Review Chapter 2: Advocating for your Loved One for additional insight). CMs help coordinate discharge for smooth transitions to the next stage of recovery, whether the survivor is discharged to a rehab facility, skilled nursing care, or their home.

Recreational Therapist: A therapist who coordinates therapeutic recreation programs to help promote social skills and leisure activities.

Respiratory Therapists: Respiratory therapists are known as either Certified Respiratory Therapists (CRT) or Registered Respiratory Therapists (RRT) depending upon their level of training. They help survivors with breathing disorders and support all aspects of a patient's breathing and lung functioning . They manage life support mechanical ventilation systems and artificial airways.

Audiologist: A healthcare professional who specializes in the evaluation and treatment of hearing and hearing loss.

Registered Dietitian: A healthcare professional who evaluates and provides for the dietary needs of individuals with special needs, including diabetics and people who need modified diets because of dysphagia (or swallowing problems).

Orthotist: A healthcare professional who makes braces and splints to strengthen or stabilize a part of the body. They commonly help survivors with walking through the use of devices like an ankle-foot orthosis (AFO) or a foot-drop stimulator (FDS).

Chaplain: A spiritual counselor who helps patients and families during crisis periods.

WHEN THE TEAM MEETS—WHAT TO EXPECT

Most rehab teams hold weekly, biweekly, or monthly meetings to discuss:

- The survivor's plan of care (i.e., what services/supports are needed)
- The survivor's progress
- Short- and long-term goals
- Intended length of stay
- Patient and family education needs
- Discharge planning

Team meetings are an opportunity for all of the medical disciplines, as well as family members, to ask questions, review what's working in the survivor's rehab treatment, what needs adjustment, and what the next steps should include. Each therapist or professional reports the present level of performance encompassing what goals have been achieved and at what level of independence. New goals are then established.

Team meetings typically last 30 minutes to an hour. Members discuss projected dates of discharge, as well as what the next care setting might be, such as a rehabilitation hospital, a skilled nursing facility, or a return home. The survivor is encouraged to attend meetings and participate to whatever degree they can. Caregivers can help a LO generate questions in anticipation of the meeting so they can be addressed with the team. You might need to advocate for your LO during meetings because the information will be technical and spoken at a pace that may be too fast for them to comprehend. For a stroke survivor, multiple speakers and a large group can make processing more difficult. After the meeting, consider reviewing the information with your LO. You may want to repeat more slowly what the clinicians have said and/or use visual aids if those help.

These team meetings are crucial to insurance adjusters who make decisions about authorizing medically necessary services. *Progress* is the key to unlocking insurance authorization. A survivor who does not make substantial progress over a period of weeks is likely to have therapy services terminated. This is why you *must* share every improvement with staff and make sure it is documented in the medical records by a nurse or therapist. "Progress" is a tricky thing because it depends on how progress is defined.

There is a difference between functional/compensatory progress and recovery. Insurance companies look for *functional progress*, what they deem "good enough" to be safe and independent, and they grade it at four different levels of assistance:

- Independent: No assistance needed
- Minimum assistance needed
- Moderate assistance needed
- Maximal assistance needed

What does *functional* really mean? In the hospital, it means the ability to do everyday tasks safely enough, using compensatory strategies. For instance, a survivor may be functional if they can get in and out of bed, use the bathroom by themselves, or get dressed, even if they have to use their *non-dominant or non-affected* side of the body or use additional tools or aids.

Physical and occupational therapists know the average hospital stay will be 8, 13, or 22 days for mild, moderate, or severely impaired stroke survivors, respectively. Therefore, they're tasked with getting people to become *functional* quickly. That way, when survivors go home, they will be as safe as possible.

At this early stage *functional* usually means relying on the unaffected, non-paralyzed side. Even if there is a small amount of movement on the affected side, that small amount won't yet be functional. In reality all therapy will be focused on *compensating for deficits* instead of the more lengthy therapeutic process of *restoring function* to the affected side.

Consequently, a survivor may be discharged or have insurance services terminated for two reasons. First, because as previously mentioned, they fail to make progress or second, the survivor's skills are deemed functional. After all, if an insurance company proves a person is functional and managing well enough, they won't likely pay for more lengthy therapy. To ensure progress and recovery continue after discharge, see Chapter 23: Powering Your Goals with "Why" Fuel.

Recovery, as opposed to functional progress, means the brain has rewired and restored sensation and movement to the affected (weak or paralyzed) side of the body. In his book, *Stronger After Stroke,* Peter G. Levine, a stroke-recovery research associate who's done stints at the Kessler Institute for Rehabilitation at the University of Cincinnati and Ohio State's B.R.A.I.N. Lab, puts it this way: "There is a downside to this focus on function.... Function does not equal recovery.... The beginning of the [brain's] rewiring process reveals itself in small amounts of movement. Small amounts of movement are considered '*non-functional*.' But small amounts of movement, while not yet providing function, are essential to the incremental process of recovery."

Levine's point is that, "when therapy focuses on "*the "good side" only, we lose the readiness period to wake up the neurons and rewire the affected, weakened side because it is ignored and not required to get better.*" According to Levine, "This process is at the core of **learned nonuse.** Learned nonuse is the result of trying and failing a movement so often, such as trying and failing to open and close a hand, that the stroke survivor believes their effort is futile, and the part of the brain that controls that movement shrinks. This, in turn, makes the movement even harder so it's done less, resulting in more brain reduction, and so on." For more information about mobility and recovery see Chapter 9: Answering Your Most Pressing "Why" Questions about Walking/Mobility.

One last note on insurance. Caregivers *must* advocate for their LOs when dealing with insurance companies, so it's essential to know two things: 1) your rights as a consumer and 2) the benefits of your insurance policy. The National Stroke Association offers excellent information about insurance as well as tips and checklists for making appeals if services are denied. Use this link to learn about your rights: *www.stroke.org/we-can-help/survivors/stroke-recovery/ lifestyle/financial/insurance-coverage-guide/insurance-appeals/ checklist*

BEST COMMUNICATION STRATEGIES WITH THE TEAM: THINK LIKE A REPORTER

Think of yourself as a reporter. Reporters take notes and pictures. Carry a notebook or some means of recording your questions, observations, and all information you receive from the doctors, nurses, and therapists. Keep an ongoing list of questions, including observations of what's improving, as well as concerns, so you're prepared when you speak to the physiatrist and the rest of the rehab team.

I recommend reviewing your notebook and highlighting your questions with a yellow marker well in advance of a meeting to insure your questions are answered. You may want to bring a recorder (your phone should come with preinstalled apps for voice recording), making sure to tell the team you'd like to record the call in order to reference anything you might not remember.

As I've said before, your perspective is critical to the team's understanding of the "holistic" picture of your LO. You paint the picture of where your LO's abilities *were* to balance where they currently are and where they're going. However, you must remember that your rehab team's perspective is valuable too. They objectively see where your LO is *now*. We must respect where a LO is *now* in order to measure progress. While it's natural to think about your LO's past and "lost" abilities, you will feel more *hope and hasten improvement* if you are in the present identifying evidence of progress moving forward.

Reader Challenge

Right now, before you forget, write down two to three questions you have for the rehab team.

***

Remember Chase, the man with the repaired aneurysm and the smeared glasses you met in the introduction? Five months prior to his aneurysm, Chase was appointed to the bench as a U.S. Superior Court judge. However, his stroke caused severe receptive and expressive aphasia, meaning he could neither understand spoken language nor could he speak. When he attempted speech, his words were incomprehensible gibberish. His understanding of language was so impaired that even the names of common objects, like "cup or comb," eluded him. Through testing and looking for *what was working*, it became clear to me that he recognized individual letters. He couldn't read, but we slowly built upon what he *could do*, until one day he read and matched ten objects (cup, comb, razor, and so on) to their printed word. Thrilled at this breakthrough, I rushed to tell his wife.

"Chase matched ten objects to their written words!" I beamed.

"Oh, hon," she said slack-faced, "we have such different baselines."

She was right. Chase was a Yale-educated Superior Court judge who routinely spoke in four-syllable words. To her, my thrilling news was a devastating confirmation of how far he was from where he'd been. But I was right too, because that's exactly where he *was*... and he *was* making progress.

Chase continued to make astounding progress as he committed to rigorous speech, occupational, and physical therapies over a period of two years. As part of his recovery, he began visiting the courtroom, first as an observer. Eventually, he transitioned from passive observer to incrementally performing tasks related to his job. When he and his therapists believed he was ready to return to work with modifications, the Commission on Judicial Performance was not as convinced. Chase had to prove his competency by submitting to intense neuropsychological testing and a thorough vetting of his skills. These tests were so demanding they would've challenged a non-brain-injured person. In the end, the Honorable Chase G. proved his competency and returned to the bench to serve as a Superior Court judge for ten more years before he retired.

BEWARE OF A RAPID DISCHARGE AND THE STROKE SURVIVOR WHO LOOKS *JUST FINE.*

Of course it's a relief and great news when a survivor is doing so well they're either not admitted to the hospital after a transient ischemic attack (TIA or mini-stroke) or they're discharged within only a few days of an actual stroke. TIAs do not cause permanent brain damage, but they are a serious warning sign that a stroke may happen in the future and that one should follow up with a physician for a full assessment. What's more, just because you don't *see* physical residual problems related to a stroke, like limb paralysis or weakness, doesn't mean the stroke survivor is at the top of their game or even out of danger.

So, why might a survivor be discharged from the hospital after only a day or two? Some patients are released because they pass every neurological screening test and appear to have no emergent nursing needs requiring hospitalization. As mentioned earlier, some people have achieved a level of *functional* ability even if they still require some assistance.

An early discharge may give everyone the impression that the stroke or TIA wasn't a serious event. This is not true. In fact, the greatest risk for one who has had a TIA is an actual stroke. Forty percent of people who have a TIA will have an actual stroke, and nearly half of all strokes occur within the first few days after a TIA. For more information see the Preface: Recognize a Stroke & Respond Immediately. Memorize the acronym FAST and seek immediate medical care if a stroke is suspected.

Brain injury is often referred to as an *invisible injury* because we can't see from the outside what's causing a person to have slower thought processing, confusion, decreased memory, difficulty with divided attention, sensory impairments, increased emotional affect, inability to interpret social cues, and/or significant fatigue. The greatest risk for those who've had an *actual* stroke is a secondary stroke, but another risk is simply doing *too much too soon*. The brain is in a fragile state of healing. "Too much too soon" might mean complex activities like driving, returning to work, or engaging in physical or mental activities that overly stress the body.

Brooke was one of those "looks great" survivors. Luckily, when Brooke experienced a sudden right-side weakening of her arm and leg, and her mouth began to feel tingly with her speech slurring, her friends recognized the classic stroke symptoms and sought medical attention. Brooke received a clot-busting drug known as tPA (tissue plasminogen activator) which halts and reverses the neurological effects of paralysis in an ischemic stroke, but *only if it's administered within three hours of the onset of the stroke symptoms.*

Brooke felt an immediate improvement in her arm and hand as the drug was administered, although she reported that symptoms reappeared to a much lesser degree later that night in the hospital. Over the next few days, Brooke appeared to recover quickly and passed every neurological and physical screening test. She was discharged after only three days of hospitalization. She was happy to return home, but was scared and uncertain. She clung to her sister's arm as she walked around her house because neither she nor her sister felt she was stable enough nor adequately informed about potential risks to walk on her own.

Brooke lived in a safe neighborhood and had the habit of leaving her home's front door not just unlocked, but wide open. Brooke also had a large group of concerned friends. During our first meeting and speech evaluation, a steady stream of visitors walked in and out of her house, oblivious to the fact an evaluation was taking place. When visitors left, Brooke spoke about the energy drain and the toll it was taking on her. Her friends were relieved to see she "looked so well," but the truth was Brooke was having attention and memory issues, not sleeping well, and experiencing slower mental processing, weakness, and incoordination in her leg and hand. She was scared and beginning to get depressed. Mostly, she was exhausted trying to entertain her friends throughout the day. When I educated both her and her family that her brain needed rest and gave them permission to limit both the amount of visitors per day and the length of time visitors came, they found the news liberating. Brooke and her sister learned to tell friends, "My brain needs a rest." This kick-started Brooke's ability to focus on her recovery and she made great progress.

Once your LO leaves the hospital and transfers home, future medical care will continue with your primary care physician, not the hospital team. Once checked out of the hospital, many survivors will never see a physiatrist again. Don't expect your primary care physician to know your LO had a stroke unless you tell them. The hospital will not communicate with outside physicians. After discharge, it's a good idea to get a referral to an outpatient physiatrist to make sure you are getting the latest and best treatments to continue recovery. See the Appendix under caregiver resources for a link to the *Evidence-Based Review of Stroke Rehabilitation* website to access the most current stroke rehabilitation therapies.

ESSENTIAL TAKEAWAYS

- You and your Loved One are the center of your rehab team.
- Focus on your LO's progress, *not* the prognosis.
- Look for and report evidence of spontaneous recovery (or *natural recovery* of function without specific effort).
- Communicate your loved one's special characteristics to the team. What makes them unique?
- Become an active participant on the team. Carry a notebook, make observations, ask questions, and record team meetings if necessary and permitted.
- Rehab teams consist of, at minimum, a Physiatrist, the head rehabilitation doctor who oversees the team and orders therapy services, an Occupational Therapist (OT); Physical Therapist (PT); Speech Therapist (ST); SW: Social Worker (SW); and a Case Manager (CM).
- Make the Case Manager your ally. Learn what insurance companies look for to authorize and continue therapy services.
- Make certain all progress is recorded in the survivor's medical records and all therapies are delivered and/or made up if missed.
- The National Stroke Association offers this link to learn about your insurance rights. *www.stroke.org/we-can-help/ survivors/stroke-recovery/lifestyle/financial/insurance-coverage-guide/insurance-appeals/checklist*
- Know the difference between functional skills and recovery.

Avoid "learned nonuse" by stimulating the neuroplastic process of recovery. See Chapter 9: Answering Your Most Pressing "Why" Questions about Walking/Mobility.

Learn about Constraint-Induced Therapy and ask if it's an option for your loved one.

- Balance the "Use It or Lose It" concept of repetition with doing too much too soon. Recognize the subtle signs of "invisible" brain injury and know when to rest. Signs include slowed processing time, difficulty managing two tasks at once (e.g., walking and talking), irritability, fatigue, and/or increased emotional affect.

- Brain healing takes time. Both activity and rest are essential.

THE SECRET SAUCE OF RECOVERING (C&S)

*Hardships often prepare ordinary people
for an extraordinary destiny.*
~ **C.S. Lewis** ~

What you and your LO need more than anything right now is perspective. Focusing on the reality of "what is" in this moment can be overwhelming, so let's look ahead, because change happens. Change is inevitable. The brain and body constantly work to achieve balance and recovery. Nothing ever stays the same.

So how *do* people recover from strokes? How do some stroke survivors become *Thrivers* and return to a meaningful life? Doctors have long researched what factors are most predictive of stroke recovery, but the results are largely inconclusive. While it seems logical to assume that the less severe a stroke is the better the outcome will be, that's not always the case. I'm often struck by how a person with minor residual impairments may view his life as ruined, whereas others who've suffered total paralysis, loss of speech and memory, talk about the gratitude and purpose they feel. Even in the presence of difficulties, Thrivers recover a life worth living.

Since it's difficult to *predict* recovery, what would happen if we looked at the exceptional survivors, the ones who were thriving, and then walked *backwards* to connect the dots? What's the *secret sauce* of a Thriver? That is, what do they think and do that makes them exceptional? I call this exceptional *recovering*, instead of recovery. As mentioned earlier, recovery is not a destination, but an ongoing, active state of being.

Here are the five non-scientific, non-evidence-based, purely anecdotal clues I've seen repeatedly be most predictive of exceptional recovering:

- An internal sense of faith and family support.
- The brain's function and abilities before the stroke (i.e., how much a person used their brain). This is not necessarily formalized schooling but curiosity and continual learning.
- A belief that the survivor is here for a reason and purpose. For instance, they may feel needed by their children, spouse, and/or family, a business, community, etc.
- A person's will, determination, and consistency of action. Athletes and others with a practice of self-discipline and familiarity with goal-setting and accomplishment come to mind.
- A reverence for the *essence* of Life.

THESE ARE THE SURVIVORS' STORIES AND BELIEFS

More than anything, faith seems to be the strongest factor in successfully recovering. It doesn't appear to matter what the *source* of faith is, just that faith is present.

What does faith look like? For agnostics and atheists, their "faith" centers on their doctors, their belief in medicine, their own determination, and their families. Other Thrivers find their faith in God, Jesus, Adonai, Buddha, Allah, Krishna, Source Energy, and so on. In my opinion, it is not the *who* or the *what* but the *action* of faith that's important. Faith, hope, and belief are not passive states of being, they're active accelerants. People don't *have* faith, they *are* faith.

I make no suggestions for any particular faith or practice. In this chapter, I'm simply relaying the stories of thriving survivors. Some stories are about those in the earlier stages of recovering, where one is actively working to restore function. Others are further along.

They might say they're "beyond recovering and simply living life," evolving as we all do, accepting and adjusting to a changed physical or cognitive function.

All however, would describe their lives as meaningful and worth waking up for in the morning. All believe they have significance, connection to others, that they contribute in some way and continue to grow. Life is not static for anyone. Everyone is continually changing.

Beyond the five factors listed above, there are always secret ingredients that make any sauce exceptional. For exceptional recovering, these are:

- Gratitude
- Humor
- Persistence
- Acceptance

THE SECRET SAUCE OF GRATITUDE

Scott was a 46-year-old engineer married for 22 years and the father of 4 girls. On a perfectly crisp, clear New Year's morning, Scott and his buddies hit the California surf. Scott's wife, Kari, had left early that morning to drive their eldest daughter to Utah for college. Scott stayed behind to care for his other 3 girls, two high schoolers and a frisky, charming, and challenging 10-year-old with Down syndrome. After surfing, Scott went to his mother's house to help move furniture. As soon as he lifted a heavy china cabinet, Scott felt nauseous and dizzy. It wasn't a New Year's hangover. Scott was Mormon and didn't drink. He thought he could shake it off and went home, but things got worse. Finally someone called 911, but by that time he was on the floor vomiting. Scott had suffered a spontaneous carotid artery dissection (or a tear inside the neck artery that goes to the brain).

When I met Scott in the hospital several weeks after his admittance, he had a scar at the base of his neck from where the ventilator had kept him alive. He was totally paralyzed on his right side, and he was wearing a helmet. Doctors had removed a portion of his skull in a procedure called a *craniectomy* to prevent his swelling brain from causing further compression and damage. The helmet protected his soft, vulnerable brain in case he fell. Scott also had a lump in his abdomen—it was his skull, otherwise known as a *bone flap*. A bone flap is often placed in the abdomen until brain swelling subsides and it can be reattached to the head.

Scott had no usable language. In fact, the sounds he uttered didn't resemble those of the English language. Their pitch, tone, and cadence sounded oddly alien.

Kari, Scott's wife, almost never left his bedside. If she wasn't attending to his needs, she was researching, praying, and managing her four daughters, including helping the eldest not only get to college, but recover all of her belongings that were stolen from their car in the hospital parking lot when they rushed to be with Scott.

Both Kari and Scott had a strong faith in God and were deeply involved with their church where Scott served as a deacon. A massive nationwide prayer circle kept vigil for Scott and his family for months.

Although Scott couldn't speak, from the moment I met him he communicated gratitude and appreciation. He would tip his head, close his eyes, and place his hand on his heart in acknowledgement. His expression was deeply heartfelt.

How did gratitude help him recover? I watched him *shape* his environment by thanking nurses, therapists, janitors, friends, and family members. Multiple times a day, Scott expressed gratitude for acts performed for him. As a result, hospital caregivers liked visiting him.

Nurses spent more time with him. They talked with him. They'd pop by his room to encourage him. They'd cheer for him as he was pushed down the hallway. Scott's gratitude made others feel better. When people feel better, they see with better eyes. Their good feelings amplified and energized his recovery. Everyone likes to be a part of a miracle.

WHATEVER YOU APPRECIATE, TO COIN A FINANCIAL TERM, *APPRECIATES.*

> Kari's journal entry, reprinted with permission:
> "*I find it strange how common laughter and smiles are within the walls of Scott's hospital room. It really is hard to focus on what has been taken away, when I am first so grateful he is alive and second to witness his strength, courage, faith, and determination as he slowly relearns skills.*"

Fred was a business executive who had a stroke in the early morning hours just after using the bathroom. His wife was accustomed to him waking and leaving the house before she awoke. After getting up, she began making the bed as usual, but when she reached Fred's side, she found him on the floor, paralyzed on his right side and unable to speak.

When I met Fred, his speech was still pretty limited, but he was getting great return of motor function on his right side. Fred was not only a business executive, but also the president of his Lions Club. He showed me a pile of get-well cards he'd received while hospitalized and pointed to the many potted plants that surrounded him. He told me how grateful he was and how he wanted to write each one a personal note of thanks. He spent many weeks painstakingly writing thank-you notes with his *new* hand that was "waking up." He wrote like a child, with poor spelling and awkward grammar. His writing looked like scribble, with ill-formed letters and odd spacing. We didn't correct those early versions; we sent them as they were.

About a month later we attended his Lions Club meeting. Despite still having mild aphasia, Fred felt ready *enough* to speak before his group. A colleague greeted him with a big hug and tears in her eyes, exclaiming how she'd cried with joy when she received his note in his own handwriting. Did she cry because of all he'd lost? No, but because that note told her he was pushing himself to grow and recover.

He'd put his ego aside and was willing to do something poorly before it got better. ("Every master is first a disaster," says David Wood, host of the Kickass Life podcast). Surprisingly, his gratitude had a ripple effect on her. She thanked him for increasing *her* gratitude for the many things she had previously ignored.

Fred eventually returned to work and resumed his presidency at the Lions Club. He also became an active member in his local stroke support group where he challenged and encouraged all survivors to make healthy lifestyle changes.

THE SECRET SAUCE OF HUMOR

Scott's quirky sense of humor was like an electric current, always on and flowing. He'd make faces and roll his eyes, saying *"Wa, wa, wa"* in a Charlie Brown voice, mocking the therapists whose enthusiastic directions came at him so fast that they sounded like a blur of sounds to him. Scott always looked for, found, or created "the funny." He once came across a picture of the *Simpsons* character, Ned Flanders, and positioned it mugshot-style next to his face, causing gales of laughter because it indeed looked like his identical twin.

Humor sometimes shows up in a simple willingness to laugh at the ridiculous. Here Superior Court Judge Chase's wife, Annie, tells her story:

"Chase and I were in his hometown driving to a place I didn't know. Chase was giving me directions; the only thing was his severe aphasia kept causing him to mix up his words for 'left' and 'right.' He'd say, 'Go left,' and I'd say, 'OK,' but as I turned left, he'd say, 'No, left!' and I'd say, 'I am going left like you told me, right?' And then he'd say, 'Right!', meaning the opposite direction. It became clear this was an impossible challenge, but we both started laughing. I finally said, 'Don't say anything, just point.' And that took care of it. It was kind of like that Abbott and Costello comedy bit, 'Who's on First?'"

The Secret Sauce of Persistence

Physical therapists go by the initials PT, but anyone who's ever worked with them knows PT is also code for "Pain and Torture." It's not intentional. Physical therapists must coax spastic or severely tight muscles into normal ranges of motion. It can be very painful and they don't do it just once. Thrivers repeat thousands of repetitive movements to achieve small gains.

Persistence is defined as *a firm or obstinate continuance in a course of action in spite of difficulty or opposition.*

At one of our speech therapy sessions, Scott was having a really tough time. His brain was fried from just having completed physical therapy. Even the simplest task, such as pointing to a cup, was going nowhere. He became increasingly frustrated, so we shifted our focus. I knew Scott was a surfer and I knew there was a program called Life Rolls On, developed by Jesse Billauer, an upcoming pro, who at 17 years of age suffered a spinal cord injury while surfing. Paralyzed from the neck down, Jesse vowed he'd surf again and that he'd help others as well.

Scott and I looked at the videos of this remarkable adaptive surfing program complete with sand wheelchairs and hundreds of volunteers helping paralyzed men and women ride the waves. He began grinning from ear to ear.

The website said there was an event in Santa Monica, California, in only four weeks. Scott was scheduled to have his bone flap (the part of his skull stored in his abdomen) returned to his head in three weeks. Not many people have to think, "Yeah, I'm going surfing in a month, but first I have to get my skull back on!"

Suddenly Scott had a new focus. Persistence no longer seemed like a grueling task, but an inspired call to action. What would he need to become and do to feel the rush of the waves again? First off, he had to believe he could do it, and second, he had to convince his doctors and wife that he was ready. He also had to get in a wetsuit. Imagine the persistence needed to squeeze into a full-length second skin when only half of his body cooperated?

Four months after Scott's life crashed in every imaginable way, he was in the ocean surfing, exactly as he had done on that fateful New Year's Day. Okay, *not exactly*. This time it took 14 people assisting him at various stages in the water, including a therapist on his surfboard, to make sure he stayed on. Yes, he was utterly exhausted, but the elation and joy Scott experienced, with his entire cheering family at the shore, was worth every ounce of persistence. He used this feeling of accomplishment as his "fuel" to drive so many other goals.

If anyone could be the poster girl for persistence, it was Kate. At the age of 31, this healthy, athletic, soon-to-be fitness trainer, wife, and mother of 2 girls, ages 18 months and 3 years old, had a double brainstem stroke that totally paralyzed her from head to toe. Because of Kate's age and apparent state of wellness, it took her doctors a long time to diagnose that she'd had a stroke. Even Kate's breathing muscles were paralyzed and required a ventilator to keep her alive.

Kate could see, hear, understand, and feel *everything*, but she had zero ability to respond. She says, "It was as if I was in a glass coffin." She couldn't even exhibit a pain reflex. Her doctors assumed she couldn't feel pain, and in effort to spare her brain from the effects of anesthesia, they performed surgical procedures *without* anesthesia. Her rare condition, known as "Locked -In Syndrome," was terrifying.

Kate's doctors initially described her condition as "vegetative" and believed her husband was delusional and in deep denial thinking she had any hope for recovery. After what seemed like an eternity, Kate and her husband discovered the one thing she could do. Kate could blink. As Kate says, "I could think and blink." To communicate, her husband used a crude alphabet board, and as he pointed to each single letter, Kate blinked once for "yes" and twice for "no." It was exhausting spelling out words. She says it took 16 blinks to say, "I love you."

Kate's fierce determination to walk out of the hospital and resume caring for and raising her babies was the fuel she used to keep her going. Kate clawed her way back to walking, talking, eating, and learning how to do everything from dressing to driving with one hand. She'd be the first to say she couldn't have survived had it not been for her husband's dogged persistence in advocating for her at every turn, insisting she receive therapy treatments and services in a rehab hospital that initially refused to treat her.

In her book, *Paralyzed but not Powerless*, her story, along with her husband's observations from the other side of the bed, give us a frank and transparent account of how her recovery affected each one in the family and how they managed their challenges, including the legal and insurance issues.

Today Kate's life is full. In her 50's she went back to school and graduated with a Bachelor's and Master's degree. She works at the Disabled Resources Center as a Job Developer and Outreach Coordinator helping others find work. Four years after her stroke, she gave a congressional speech urging congress to fund research for stroke and heart disease. She continues speaking professionally about healing and recovery after stroke.

THE SECRET SAUCE OF ACCEPTANCE

According to Elisabeth Kubler-Ross, a psychiatrist whose groundbreaking work on death, dying and loss identified five stages of grief. These include: Denial, Anger, Bargaining, Depression and Acceptance.

Acceptance is often confused with the notion of being in agreement or "okay" with what has happened to a person. This is not the case. People who *thrive* accept that a stroke has happened, but they don't necessarily view it as a static state. Thrivers learn to adjust to a changed and changing condition. They learn to experience a new norm. They discover that more stress comes from resisting what happened and focusing on the past. *They also discover that more growth and progress come from accepting where they are and moving toward the best they can be.* It's not an overnight process. It comes as a result of going through the four other stages identified, but glimmers of acceptance can show up even in some of the earlier stages.

Scott's wife shared another of her journal entries:
"Even when Scott mouths and gestures 'Why God, why?' He isn't angry... more curious. It helps to not focus on why. Just to say it sucks and to think about how blessed we've been during this journey. Scott is alive. He is already 28 days into this and has exceeded all the doctor's predictions. Every day Scott makes steps forward toward regaining what he's lost. Our family has been blessed with support and love."

Another Thriver, Howard, describes coming out of his "vegetable state" and spending a month in the hospital engaged in rigorous PT, OT, and ST. In the midst of his own recovery, he says, he never struggled with acceptance. "It just happened. I just accepted this was my new life." When asked if he'd always had such a resilient attitude, he chuckled. "No, I lost a job once and went into a deep depression."

He couldn't explain why he so readily accepted the significant life changes he faced, but he said, "I remember being in my hospital bed; my roommate was groaning in pain, but unable to activate his call button. I asked if he wanted me to call for help. When the nurse arrived and helped him, I suddenly felt like I'd made a contribution. This feeling of being able to help someone else gave me purpose. I discovered that when I helped others, I didn't have time to notice my own problems.

I started volunteering to speak to the 'new guys' who had strokes. My speech therapist, who was also a professor at a university, asked me to speak to his students to get a *real-life* understanding of aphasia. Eventually I volunteered at two different hospitals. Now I volunteer at the VA Hospital. It's not that I have an 'important' job, really, anyone could do it, but I feel that even my menial jobs make a difference."

"Acceptance" comes in time and with varying levels of meaning. Regardless of whether one has a brain injury or not, we all must face many life challenges and changes. The reality is we can only *be where we are* at any moment in time. It may be useful to know and say, *"I am where I am, but in every moment, with every thought and feeling, I can choose where I'm going."*

ESSENTIAL TAKEAWAYS

Exceptional *recovering* includes five factors:

- An internal sense of faith and family support.
- The brain's function and abilities before the stroke, (i.e., how much a person used their brain). This is not necessarily formalized schooling but curiosity and active continual learning.
- A belief that a person is here for a reason and purpose. For instance, they may feel needed by their children, spouse, and/or family, a business, community, etc.
- A person's will, determination, and consistency of action.
- A reverence for the *essence* of Life.

Gratitude, Humor, Persistence, and Acceptance are the secret ingredients in the sauce of exceptional recovering.

You are only *where you are* at any moment in time. It helps to know and say, *"I am where I am, but in every moment, with every thought and feeling, I can choose where I'm going."*

CHANGE YOUR LANGUAGE, SHAPE YOUR LIFE (C&S)

Words don't describe our reality, they shape it.
~ Tony Robbins ~

We are what we think and we are what we speak. Part of your successful recovery as either a caregiver or survivor is influenced by the language that you use.

So often we are either unconscious or careless about our word choices. When I trained with Tony Robbins, one of the world's most renowned and influential personal development gurus, he asked us to make a list of the emotions we felt at least once a week. Although there are 3,000 words to describe emotions, most people reported habitually feeling about 5 good feelings with the rest being negative. In fact, 90% of the people wrote down an average of a dozen feelings and more than half of those words described negative feelings. Robbins described this as a universal response he has seen over more than two decades, with audience sizes ranging from 2,000 to 30,000 people worldwide. With so much emphasis on negative emotion, is it any wonder depression is on the rise?

The question is do we feel bad or worse *because* of the *words* we choose? Robbins examined the language patterns of different people and how those patterns either magnified or softened an emotion. He found words like "furious" or "enraged" had a different tone than "peeved" or "upset" and that each had different physiological outcomes as well. He proved words don't just describe our reality, they actually shape it.

When I met Toby she was 10 days into her stroke recovery. She was hospitalized briefly, but because she was medically stable, could walk and understand language, she'd been discharged.

Toby had an imposing physical presence, a stern, tough, no-nonsense attitude, with a hair-trigger temper belied by the softness of her light blue eyes. Although Toby had no physical challenges, she had severe reading impairments and a very limited ability to speak or express herself. One thing she made clear, though, was that she was adamant about living on her own in the company of her two cats. The question I had to help answer was, *Would she be safe?*

Toby was an insulin-dependent diabetic who gave herself injections multiple times a day. She also had extremely high blood pressure, the unfortunate source of her stroke. She left the hospital with several new medications and written instructions for her changed insulin dosages. While I assessed her ability to read the prescription labels and match the dosing directions, she launched into a torrent of swear words followed by a verbal self-lashing: "I'm stupid. I'm an idiot. I'm a jerk. I can't read." This was not a one-time event. Toby routinely berated herself. It was painful to be present for such abuse.

"What would you do if a doctor called you an idiot?" I asked.

"I'd say, 'You're an idiot,'" she responded, and yet she failed to see how her words were damaging her.

While my "pain" at listening to her was momentary, Toby was speaking her way into a constant state of stress and declining health. Her blood pressure numbers soared to dangerous levels and her glucose readings were so erratic she was at high risk for a recurrent stroke.

Were her words making her sicker?

Yes, according to Dr. Andrew Newberg. In his book with coauthor Mark Robert Waldman, *Words Can Change Your Brain*, he says, "A single word has the power to influence the expression of genes that regulate physical and emotional stress."

While Toby might be an extreme example, most of us could use some language upgrades. For instance, a stroke patient is often referred to as a stroke *victim*. Think about it. What is the picture you conjure up when you hear the word *victim* versus *survivor* versus *warrior* versus *thriver*?

What about the countless patients, doctors, and therapists who refer to the side of the body paralyzed by the stroke as the "*bad* side," with the innocent intention that it's easier to identify than saying right, left, or affected? But *bad* implies something to avoid, reject, and neglect. If something's *bad,* we get angry at it and want it to go away.

Many stroke survivors feel separate from their bodies. They reject them, feel shame and disappointment. As a result, it requires both a language upgrade and a mindset shift to integrate the body into wholeness.

SIMPLE LANGUAGE HACKS AND MAKEOVERS

I suggest that survivors call their weaker side their "new" side or their "sassy" side. (After all, a common acronym for the stroke-affected side is SAS!). This idea of *newness* suggests the opportunity the survivor has to grow. Growth requires attention and nurturing. *Sassy* feels spunky and playful.

What may seem like a silly game of semantics is actually a powerful mindset change. Shifting from "bad" to "sassy" or "new" can send strong signals throughout the entire body to promote healing. Wouldn't you be more curious about your "sassy" side, what it needs, and how it's progressing? The sassy side needs love and appreciation to integrate. Whatever we appreciate *appreciates,* meaning it rises in value. This includes appreciation for one's body.

I encourage survivors to look at their sassy new sides and talk to them, expressing all their feelings, including asking for forgiveness for not paying attention to them, or for being mad at them, or for hating them so much they wanted to disconnect from them. I suggest that people speak lovingly to the body part(s) they've neglected and to ask the part(s) what they need and want to successfully integrate.

No, this is not "traditional" therapy, but it is based in the science of how thoughts change brain chemistry and influence healing. Dr. Bruce Lipton, a stem cell biologist and the author of numerous books including *The Biology of Belief,* is responsible for groundbreaking research performed at Stanford University's School of Medicine between 1987 and 1992. His discoveries challenged the established scientific view that genes controlled life. He demonstrated that it was the cell's *environment* that controlled the cell's behavior and physiology and influenced whether a gene turns on or off. His work foreshadowed the field of epigenetics, which studies what makes some genes turn on or express and other genes turn off or suppress, without a change in the DNA sequence.

Dr. Lipton stated, "The blood's chemistry is largely impacted by the chemicals emitted from your brain. So this means that your perception of any given thing, at any given moment, can influence the brain chemistry, which, in turn, affects the environment where your cells reside and controls their fate. **In other words, your thoughts and perceptions have a direct and overwhelmingly significant effect on cells**" (emphasis mine).

The medical literature is full of other studies showing the benefits of positive mind-body suggestions. For instance, positive suggestions given to patients during surgery resulted in those patients having decreased blood loss, decreased complications, and decreased length of hospitalizations as well as reduced post-operative pain.

Positive, loving language activates the *parasympathetic nervous system,* commonly referred to as the relaxation response, which in turn, activates the immune system. It creates a healthy environment in which cells can thrive. Most importantly, positive language doesn't trigger the stress response, which causes a cascade of hormones that suppress the body's powers of healing.

How does this relate to therapy and recovery? We are responsible for the suggestions, by way of language and thought, that we give ourselves and allow others to give us.

"Up with the good, down with the *bad.*" This is the familiar cue given to help a survivor remember which leg they should lead with when going up or down the stairs. While this phrase is catchy and memorable, it reinforces "bad."

What if we shifted our language to say, "Up with the good, down with the *new or sassy*"? Do you feel the energetic shift? If we want to move towards wholeness and integration, we need to be vigilant and purposeful about the words we choose.

How about the *handicap placard*? Ugh. Every time I hear this, I am reminded of limitation. I refer to it as the *VIP pass*. It's the best parking in town. Before heading out the door with a patient, I ask, "Did you remember to bring your VIP pass?"

"Let's get you into your diaper," healthcare professionals and caregivers may say. I cringe when I hear this, as if it's not humbling enough to have everyone know your private business. Adults wear *briefs*, not diapers.

If we're elevating our consciousness about words, what about answering those standard seemingly innocuous questions like, "How are you doing?"

So often I hear people either give a laundry list of complaints in response or answer with what they think is a positive statement, "I can't complain." But what "I can't complain" really says is, "I want to complain and I'm frustrated that I can't." Is it ever appropriate to list your complaints? Of course it is, when speaking with your medical team as you look for solutions. But for general small talk, practice making this phrase automatic: "It's not easy, but I'm getting better every day."

Wait, why shouldn't we say, "It's *hard*, but I am getting better every day?"

The word "hard" reinforces a negative and difficult state. We want to align our brains with healing and since the brain doesn't directly process negatives, it omits hearing the word "not" and instead only hears "easy," which it associates with "getting better each day." In other words, this mental mindset aligns with healing. The brain hears, "It's not easy, but I'm getting better every day."

Yes, you may mock the simplicity of this, or outright reject its significance, but one small change can shift the tone of recovery. Our thoughts are powerful. They create our feelings, which direct our actions, which create our results. And now we also know our thoughts can actually change the chemistry of our brains and our blood.

ESSENTIAL TAKEAWAYS

- Language doesn't just describe your reality, it shapes it.
- Choose the words that support the outcomes you want.
- You and your LO are warriors and thrivers, not just survivors and certainly not victims.
- Your handicap placard is your VIP pass.
- Your affected side is your "NEW" side or your Sassy side—get curious about it.
- Whatever you appreciate *appreciates* and gains value.
- Make this phrase automatic: "It's not easy, but I'm getting better every day."
- Thoughts can actually change the chemistry of our brains and our blood.

ANSWERING YOUR MOST PRESSING "WHY" QUESTIONS

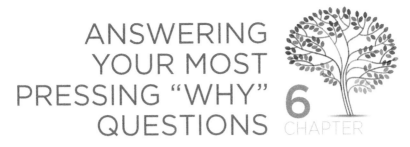

A PRELUDE (C)

When I had all the answers the questions changed.
~ Brida, Paulo Coelho ~

WHY DID THIS HAPPEN?

While this is an important and necessary question, because 80% of strokes are actually preventable, that "why" is best answered by your doctor. In general, strokes occur because of factors like genetics, stress, diet, exercise, medications, blood pressure, and lifestyle. See the infographic on how to Recognize a Stroke and respond FAST at the beginning of the book. For an infographic on how to Prevent a Stroke, see the end of the book.

What many of you are really asking and want to know is *how* will the stroke affect my LO? More importantly, you want to know … what *will make things better? When will things improve?*

You will hear a recurrent theme throughout this book:

> **NO TWO STROKES ARE ALIKE.**
> **Every stroke is different because every brain**
> **is uniquely different.**

This is not a cop-out for avoiding specific answers or strategies. In fact you will find many specific answers to your pressing questions in the next several chapters, but the reality is, there is not a one-size-fits-all approach to answering questions about or treating stroke.

THE IMPACT OF THE BRAIN'S STRUCTURE ON STROKE RECOVERING

The human brain looks very much like a walnut and is composed of two parts: a right hemisphere and a left hemisphere connected by a bridge called the *corpus callosum*. Each hemisphere is thought to process information differently. See the image below for more details.

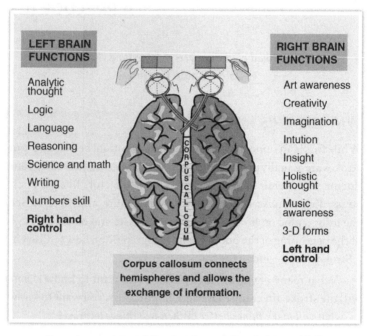

Top down view of the brain and the right and left hemisphere functions

When you see paralysis or weak muscles on one side of the body, the damage is coming from the opposite (or *contralateral*) side of the brain. In other words, the left hemisphere of the brain controls the right side of the body, and the right hemisphere controls the left side of the body.

Within the hemispheres are specialized lobes of the brain responsible for motor and sensory functions. The following image will help you see how the brain is typically mapped for location of different functions.

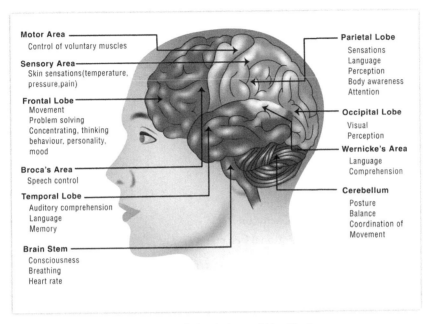

Motor Area
Control of voluntary muscles

Sensory Area
Skin sensations(temperature, pressure,pain)

Frontal Lobe
Movement
Problem solving
Concentrating, thinking
behaviour, personality,
mood

Broca's Area
Speech control

Temporal Lobe
Auditory comprehension
Language
Memory

Brain Stem
Consciousness
Breathing
Heart rate

Parietal Lobe
Sensations
Language
Perception
Body awareness
Attention

Occipital Lobe
Visual
Perception

Wernicke's Area
Language
Comprehension

Cerebellum
Posture
Balance
Coordination of
Movement

Functions of the Lobes of the Brain

Now that you can visualize the areas of the brain and their functions, let's move on to answering your "Why?", "When?", and "How to Make it Better?" questions. Regrettably, many of the answers to "When?" include those two uncertain words: *It depends.*

While the MRI's and CT scans will answer your "what" and "where" questions about the location and damage of your LO's stroke, most of your "whys" will come from what you observe when you look at or listen to your LO as they try to function in their new, post-stroke life.

As a caregiver, I encourage you to learn as much as possible, but I also caution you not to take on too many roles. Caregivers have enough added stressors and daily tasks—you don't need to become a therapist as well. If you try to assume that role, it may put more stress on both of you and likely damage, not enhance, your relationship. For the same reason spouses generally shouldn't teach one another to drive or play golf, strive to be a lover and a friend, not a therapist. You can celebrate successes, facilitate and coordinate services, and reinforce therapy goals instead.

In the next five chapters, you'll get some answers that will help sharpen your skills in asking more precise questions of your care providers.

So, how will a stroke *affect* your LO? The most commonly asked questions fall into five main areas:

- Communication
- Eating/Swallowing
- Walking/Mobility
- Memory/Cognition
- Social/Emotional Behaviors

Regardless of the area of concern, though, be encouraged that these three *practices* can make anything and everything better:

- Ask questions and become informed.
- Look for and celebrate evidence of all signs of progress.
- Practice love, appreciation, and find humor whenever and wherever you can.

ESSENTIAL TAKEAWAYS

- No two strokes are alike. Every stroke is different because every brain is uniquely different.
- Learn which parts of the brain are responsible for various bodily functions to better understand a survivor's behaviors.
- Caregivers should avoid taking on the role of a *therapist*. Instead, a caregiver can facilitate and coordinate services, reinforce therapy goals, and be a supportive fan.
- Ask questions. Become informed.
- Look for and celebrate evidence of all signs of progress.
- Practice love, appreciation, and find humor whenever and wherever you can.

COPING WITH COMMUNICATION CHALLENGES

7

ANSWERING YOUR MOST PRESSING "WHY" QUESTIONS ABOUT SPEECH (C)

To communicate through silence is a link
between the thoughts of man.
~ Marcel Marceau ~

Imagine your room filled with filing cabinets, packed with your most important documents. Now imagine that a crane comes through, shaking and emptying the contents of each and every one. Hundreds of thousands of papers scatter. Now, in the resulting mess, picture trying to locate just one very crucial document quickly.

That's what *aphasia* (ah-FAY-zhuh) is like. The words are not exactly lost, but finding and retrieving them is a monumental task. That's the physical part of aphasia; but "losing" the ability to communicate is tantamount to losing one's connection to the world.

- Why can't my LO talk? What is aphasia, and does it affect intelligence?
- How can I communicate with someone who doesn't speak or understand me?
- How long does aphasia last?
- Is aphasia curable? Treatable?
- How is aphasia treated?
- Why does my LO sound drunk?

WHY CAN'T MY LO TALK? WHAT IS APHASIA, AND DOES IT AFFECT INTELLIGENCE?

Aphasia is an acquired communication disorder that impairs a person's ability to process language in the areas of speaking and understanding. Often reading and writing skills are also impaired. Aphasia does *not* impact intelligence. Instead, having aphasia is like suddenly being dropped into a country whose language you don't speak. Your intelligence remains the same, but you can't communicate using language.

Aphasia comes from Greek words that mean "a loss of language"—literally the words are irretrievable (but not necessarily gone). The formerly automatic neural pathways that made speech effortless have been damaged and shut down like a major highway that has an impassable road. Much like a repair crew, the brain works to create alternate paths to retrieve words, but with aphasia, this process is often slow or even inaccessible, causing a total breakdown in communication.

There are five types of aphasia with very different characteristics. They are generally categorized by either being *fluent* or *nonfluent*. Most often, though, you will simply hear the term "aphasia" used to broadly describe a communication difficulty.

TYPES AND SEVERITY OF
APHASIA

LEAST
SEVERE

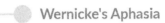

Anomic Aphasia

Word finding difficulties especially for nouns and verbs. Grammar may be fluent, but speech output is full of vague and frustrated circumlocutions. (Ex. the thing you know for watering) may mean "hose." They understand speech well. Word finding difficulties seen in writing.

FLUENT

Wernicke's Aphasia

Speech is fluent, however far from normal. Often sentences lack content. Jargon and neologisms (made up words) appear. Comprehension is impaired. Reading and writing are often severely impaired

Mixed Non-Fluent Aphasia

Sparse and limited speech resembling Broca's, but with more limited comprehension. Reading and writing skills are at an elementary level.

NON
FLUENT

Broca's Aphasia

Speech output is severely reduced to short utterances of < 4 words. Vocabulary is limited. Halting and effortful speech. Comprehension and reading may be intact. Limited Writing.

MOST
SEVERE

Global Aphasia

Most severe. Few recognizable words. Severely impaired comprehension. Unable to read or write. Global aphasia may be seen immediately after stroke and may improve if damage is not too extensive.

Types and Severity of Aphasia

In general, with nonfluent aphasia, speech is slow and effortful and may be limited to nouns or a few key words. Survivors complain, "It's hard to get the words out." This causes great frustration for both the speaker and the listener. The person with nonfluent aphasia often has intact comprehension or receptive language, meaning that they *understand* what's being said.

What is confounding to everyone, and most of all to the survivor, is that sometimes the survivor may speak with relative ease, yet at other times they struggle, especially if the situation is novel, highly stressful, includes multiple new people, if they feel pressured for time, or if they are fatigued.

Emotional situations can either enhance or diminish a survivor's ease in speaking. Sometimes strong emotions can actually *aid* in language fluency. That was the case for Lucy.

> Lucy was a 62-year-old woman who had nonfluent aphasia. It was hard for her to say single words, much less use a full sentence. Her speech, however, was steadily improving, and she found that writing the first letter of a word often triggered her ability to say the word, but what turned out to be her best speech therapy? Being a backseat driver while her elderly mother drove. Lucy's emotions were on high as she directed her mother, "Turn there! Too far, turn around. It's the wrong wrong! Oh, boy!"

Strong emotions can also bring about great fluency with curse words, even for people who've never used them before. Rob, an elderly, refined gentleman, detested his son's wife. While he couldn't recall her name, calling her "the bitch woman" rolled right off his tongue.

Fluent aphasia (or Wernicke's aphasia) on the other hand means that a survivor has relative ease in speaking. *Expressive language* refers to what a survivor says either verbally, or in some cases through pointing, writing, drawing, or gesturing. A person with Wernicke's aphasia has lots of speech; it just may not make sense. In the hospital, a person with Wernicke's aphasia may be easily mistaken for *not* having communication problems, because at first glance, they mostly sound and look "normal." They have normal articulation, intonation, and melody, and may carry on automatic conversations ("Hi, how are you?") with relative ease. But within a short time, you can tell something's not quite right. Their word order seems random, and they may make up words (*neologisms*) or use jargon. Their language is often referred to as "word salad."

> Danny, a retired college professor, is a perfect example.
> During a speech assessment, I asked, "Danny, what do you do with a fork?"
> Danny's response: "A fleeberjab is most astoundingly the pickle plate and we have to have it for the dinnerus."

HOW CAN I COMMUNICATE WITH SOMEONE WHO DOESN'T SPEAK OR UNDERSTAND ME?

For starters, at least initially, the caregiver will bear the load of the communication interaction with your LO. The good news though is you're equipped for this task even if you don't know it. It *is* possible to understand someone even when very few words or none at all are exchanged. Think back to a time in your life when, without words, you intuited what was being communicated.

Can you recall a time when you:

- Cared for an infant
- Watched a pantomime and understood a whole story without a single word
- Visited a foreign country and didn't speak the language or communicated with someone who didn't speak English

To be clear, the Person with Aphasia (PWA) is not an infant. This first example is only used to remind you that you *already have some skills communicating when language is lacking*. At some point in your life, you have been attuned to the whole realm of communication. In that moment, you looked and listened to and for every possible clue, verbal and nonverbal, as well as the contextual clues for what else was happening. This led you to understand what was being communicated. Did you get it right every time? No, but *no one gets it right all the time, even when language and speech are fully intact.* Not so surprisingly, the number one complaint in **all** relationships is communication, *whether aphasia is present or not.*

WHY YOU CAN UNDERSTAND EVEN IF THE WORDS AREN'T PRESENT

Communication is made up of:
7% words
55% body language
38% vocal signals

Capitalize on your understanding by looking at your LO's body language and listening to their tone of voice to aid in understanding.

You make communication better by working to understand your LO—not just their words, but the whole of their communication.

Speech therapists may give you strategies for each specific communication problem. There are also a number of apps and therapeutic programs to aid in recovery of speech (see suggested resources in the Appendix), but regrettably, because of the complexity of language and the impossibility of controlling or manipulating the words that come or don't come out of one's mouth, there is no one surefire recipe for success.

Chase's wife, Annie, said it was "months" in the hospital before she realized Chase wasn't really talking. It wasn't that she was in denial or lacked observational skills; she was the executive director of marketing and communications at a prestigious university. It was that she was attuned to Chase. "I *always* understood him," Annie said. "It wasn't until we were in a group sharing session, where I listened to him trying to talk about a photograph, that I actually realized he struggled to say real words."

HOW LONG DOES APHASIA LAST?

Regrettably, no one can predict this. Typically one sees the most amount of recovery of language in the first three months after a stroke; *however,* with repeated practice and engagement, survivors can and do continue to improve throughout their lifetime. "Use It or Lose It" applies to speech communication just as much as it does to the recovery of motor function.

Approximately 30% of all strokes result in a person having aphasia. The impact of this communication challenge may cause frustration for both the survivor and the caregiver. Over time, it can significantly impact social relationships and lead to isolation for both the caregiver and the survivor. Learning alternative communication strategies as well as forming new relationships will improve your wellbeing. For a discussion of friendships and social relationships after a stroke, see Chapter 25: Getting Your Life Back and the Appendix for support group resources.

IS APHASIA CURABLE? TREATABLE?

Aphasia is not curable, per se, but it *is* treatable to varying degrees. One may even see aphasia symptoms resolve or disappear spontaneously as a survivor recovers and the brain heals. Treating persistent aphasia requires consistent effort and may result in the use of compensatory strategies to augment or even supplement missing language skills.

HOW IS APHASIA TREATED?

A multitude of therapy techniques and treatment approaches exist for aphasia, depending on the type of aphasia the person has.

This chapter will share some of the many treatment modalities available. Most importantly, you should learn as much about your LO's specific type of aphasia or communication impairment as possible so you can investigate the best possible treatment options and resources as well as where therapy can take place.

The biggest game changer in accessibility to speech therapy, long after outpatient therapy stops, is the advent of technology. Online resources and apps bring speech therapy to the survivor's home, allowing more frequent practice time and connection to others at a more affordable price. Many resources are free or low-cost, and some may even be reimbursable by Medicare. See the Appendix for speech therapy resources, including a link to a downloadable e-book about aphasia and communication tips.

ESSENTIAL ANSWERS: Best Tips for Caregivers for Aiding Communication

- Seek to understand your LO.
- Believe you will find a way to understand.
- Make communication interactions as relaxed as possible.
- Decrease stress by allowing your LO more time for processing information.
- Accept and learn to interpret verbal attempts. Allow for imperfection.
- Remember, your LO is an adult, and every communicative interaction should reflect that level of dignity.
- Slow down communication. Use shorter sentences and make gestures that match your words.
- Use proper names (e.g., Sam or Mary) versus pronouns (e.g., he, she, they). Pronouns can get mixed up in longer exchanges, and the person with aphasia (PWA) can get lost.

- Keep face-to-face communication so you both can observe more nonverbal cues.
- Provide pencil and paper. Sometimes a PWA can self-cue by writing either a single letter or word. A PWA might alternatively draw a picture, and you can guess from there.

Are you thinking these strategies seem obvious and overly simplistic? Remember that *simple* is not always *easy*. I often see communication breakdowns *simply* because people fail to use *simple* strategies.

The biggest mistake you can make is to depend solely on your LO to complete the communication. Work collaboratively to achieve understanding, but respect your LO's need for time to process. Avoid filling in words or guessing too quickly.

WHY DOES MY LO SOUND DRUNK?

Slurred "drunk" speech related to aphasia is a result of *paresis* (weakened muscles) or paralyzed muscles. Paresis may also result in drooling or dribbling food from the mouth. A person may be cognitively intact, but have the motor impairment called *dysarthria*. Regrettably, a person with dysarthria may be misjudged as being drunk, on drugs, or mentally deficient. This can lead to problems in the future, especially as related to driving, should the person be pulled over by a police officer. See suggestions for averting this problem in Chapter 26 Driving & Working. There are two main motor impairments of speech but they are quite different.

Dysarthria (**dis-ARTH-ree-uh**): With dysarthria, the oral muscles are weak or paralyzed and can't form words. The tongue has eight muscles. The lips and cheeks also have muscles that help with speech production, chewing, and moving food into a ball (or *bolus*) in preparation for swallowing. Think about what it feels like to have a massive Novocain™ injection at the dentist—a decreased or absent sensation and weak or paralyzed muscles in and around your mouth. When these muscles are weak or paralyzed, a person may slur words, drool, dribble food from their mouth, trap food in the pockets of the cheeks, and have trouble swallowing because they can't form food into a ball and push it toward the back of the mouth.

Apraxia (ay-PRAK-see-uh): In this condition, the oral muscles are strong, but they've lost the ability to *volitionally sequence* motor movements. The keyword is volitionally. A person may automatically demonstrate the ability to perform a task, but not upon command. Apraxia may occur orally (e.g., a person may stick out his tongue when asked to blow a kiss), verbally (e.g., a person may not be able to repeat words because he cannot volitionally match the sequence of sounds to make words), or it can occur in limbs (e.g., a person may comb his hair in response to being asked to pantomime brushing his teeth.) Limb apraxias make it hard for a PWA to use gestures to augment their missing speech simply because they can't get their limbs to do what they want even if they are able to conceptualize an intended gesture.

ESSENTIAL ANSWERS: What Makes It Better

For dysarthria, encourage your LO to use and learn the steps in the acronym BLEPS:

- Breathe from the diaphragm
- Louder volume
- Exaggerate articulators (i.e., lips and tongue)
- Pace speech. Take a break and breathe between a string of three or four naturally grouped words.
- Slow down

For apraxia, try stimulating mirror neurons.

Read my lips! If the problem is apraxia, which is not a muscle weakness, but a motor sequencing disorder, and your LO cannot sequence the tongue and lip movements to make the appropriate sounds, you can record a close-up video of just your lips, saying the word over and over. Do this slowly (but not too slowly) and clearly. This is known to stimulate mirror neurons in the survivor's brain so that they can learn to synchronize body movements with those presented to produce the sounds/words. This type of therapy is very useful and is called VAST: Visual Assisted Speech Therapy.

For more speech therapy resources, home apps, and useful programs, see the Appendix under the Speech header.

WHAT YOUR LO WITH APHASIA WANTS *YOU TO* KNOW

Even if a PWA can make their needs and wants known, that is only a fraction of the whole of communication. Being able to comment, disagree, share ideas, ask questions, and use language to deepen intimacy is a fundamental part of being human. A person with aphasia (PWA) may experience feelings of frustration, isolation, loss, and unworthiness. The PWA may become easily annoyed because they think they're saying something clearly and it's the listener who's dense and not understanding. These are just a few things a PWA wants others to know:

- I am an adult, not a child. Speak to me like an adult.
- My intellect and hearing are *not* impaired.
- I need more time to process and respond.
- Be patient. I am scared, hurt, and trying my best.
- Be honest if you don't understand.
- Use humor, *not* sarcasm.
- You will probably need to repeat things many times.
- Make sure you have my attention. Don't speak to me from another room.
- Tell me if you are changing the subject of conversation.

Beyond using these daily strategies to help make communication easier, there are many types of speech therapy specifically for the survivor. An evaluation by a speech therapist will help you determine the best approach to choose. "The Aphasia Therapy Guide" by Dr. G. Albyn Davis describes the two categories of therapy. His guide can be found on website for the National Aphasia Association: *www. aphasia.org/aphasia-resources/aphasia-therapy-guide/.*

He states that therapeutic approaches fall into two categories:

- **Impairment-Based Therapy:** Working on specific listening, speaking, reading, and writing skills.
- **Communication-Based Therapy:** Whole/functional communication using whatever means are available to communicate a message.

Within these categories, however, there are a multitude of treatments, some of which are listed on the next page. Because every brain is different (yeah, you've heard that before), there is not a one-size-fits-all approach to recovering language. Relearning language for a PWA is an odd mix of having a foundation of language, but still relearning at the most basic level, which can sometimes making the PWA feel like a child.

As previously stated, we must strive to respect the dignity of the adult while providing them with the most simplistic relearning strategies. Most likely, hospital therapy will center on both impairment-based training (working on listening, understanding skills and speaking) as well as functional holistic training to make needs understood.

There are three things you should know about any therapy:

- Therapy should always be survivor-driven. That means it must reflect a survivor's unique goals and interests. It must matter to them. Otherwise there won't be any intrinsic motivation to push them forward.
- Therapy *should* change over time as a survivor improves.
- Therapy can combine both impairment training and functional communication techniques.

TYPES OF SPEECH THERAPY

This is a brief overview of the many types of therapy approaches available. Discuss these and other options with a speech therapist. The list is not exhaustive, nor does it suggest that any specific type is superior to another.

Impairment-Based Therapies

- **Melodic Intonation Therapy (MIT):** The treatment approach is based on the observation that some aphasics can *sing* words they can't speak. This treatment uses elements of rhythm and melody to improve verbal expression beginning with two-to three-syllable phrases up to full sentences.

- **Constraint-Induced Therapy (CIT):** Developed by Edward Taub, Ph.D., first as a physical therapy treatment for recovery from paralysis, this therapy relies on three principles:

  1. **Constraint**: Avoid compensation. No gestures, no drawing, no facial expressions, or alternative communication devices are allowed.

  2. **Forced Use**: Communicate only by talking. Taub's therapy allows only specific verbal words to be used and repeated. The program builds on specific phrases and expands to sentences.

  3. **Massed Practice**: Intensive therapy with a short overall duration. Therapy sessions are typically three hours a day for two weeks.

- **VNeST Therapy: Verb Network Strengthening Treatment (VNeST Therapy):** The idea is that by focusing on verbs, which require connections to nouns, one can strengthen all the words in the mental network around the verb. Targeting a variety of words helps one think of the words faster and more independently. Intentionally, VNeST therapy does not use picture cards. It is meant to activate the mental images and words in the brain and encourage flexible thought.

- **Naming Therapy with Cueing Hierarchies:** This treatment combines picture naming with supported cues, including semantic (similar words), phonemic (the initial sound of the word), and orthographic (written first letter).

- **VAST™**: Speech-impaired individuals watch close-up videos of the mouth and practice speaking with the prerecorded videos. The simultaneous combination of visual, auditory, and, in some cases, written cues, allows these individuals to mirror the movements needed to produce speech. Useful for apraxia and aphasia.

- **Computer-Based Treatment:** Touchscreen tablets and/or apps target various language needs and generate data about a person's progress.
- **Multimodal Therapy:** This treatment focuses on effective communication strategies using nonverbal and alternative augmentative communication (AAC) with or without a tablet such as an iPad that may offer spoken speech.
- **Visual Action Therapy (VAT):** Not to be confused with VAST, this treatment is used most often with people who have *global aphasia*, the most severe type affecting all modalities of communication, including speaking, understanding, reading, and writing. VAT incorporates a 12-step training hierarchy beginning with tracing objects, then matching objects, then pantomiming gestures for visible objects, then pantomiming gestures for absent objects.

Communication-Based Therapies

- **Life Participation Approach:** Typically this therapy takes place at home and in the community. It focuses on long-term management of aphasia, placing the life concerns of the PWA at the center for decision making.
- **Promoting Aphasics' Communicative Effectiveness (PACE):** This program is designed to improve conversational skills. The clinician and PWA take turns sending and receiving messages. Participants share information about a picture that is hidden from their listener. Participants are encouraged to use whatever communicative strategy they can.
- **Conversational Coaching:** A treatment designed to teach verbal and nonverbal communication strategies to the PWA and their primary partners (e.g., spouse or children). This can include gestures, drawing, cueing,

and summarizing information practiced in scripted conversations.

- **AphasiaScripts:** Written scripts are created for functional social situations. The person with aphasia practices using the script until they feel comfortable using it in daily life situations. A virtual therapist provides help for the PWA.
- **Supported Communication Intervention:** Communicative confidence is enhanced through community support groups. Volunteers are trained to engage in real conversations with persons who have aphasia. Similar therapies go by different names including "conversation therapy" or "scaffolded conversations."

For a list of speech therapy resources, including apps and programs, see the Appendix.

ESSENTIAL ANSWERS: What Makes It Better

- Seek first to *understand*. Assume you will eventually understand.
- Aphasia does not affect intelligence. It is not curable, but it is treatable. Improvement can continue throughout a person's lifetime, but it takes persistence and consistency.
- There are two categories of rehabilitative therapies, which are often integrated: Impairment-Based and Functional Communication-Based.
- Reducing stress around speaking is fundamental to improving your LO's speech.
- Caregivers, family, and friends should implement five basic strategies when communicating with a survivor:
  1. Maintain eye contact when conversing.
  2. Check for understanding.
  3. Give adequate time for your LO to respond.
  4. Use a pleasant tone of voice and facial gestures.
  5. Repeat questions or instructions as necessary, and add visual prompts and cues if needed.

ANSWERING YOUR MOST PRESSING
"WHY" QUESTIONS ABOUT
EATING/
SWALLOWING (C)

8
CHAPTER

Food is not just eating energy.
It's an experience.
~ Guy Fieri ~

E ating is one of the greatest joys of life and an important social activity that connects people. When normal swallowing is affected by a stroke, it can result in more than just a crisis of nutrition or potential infection. At the extreme, difficulties with eating, drinking, and/or swallowing can lead a person to isolate himself. According to the American Stroke Association, up to 65% of stroke patients may experience *dysphagia* (DIS-fay-zhuh), a swallowing disorder. While dysphagia may be present immediately after stroke, over time and with intervention, many stroke survivors completely recover and resume their ability to eat normally and enjoy the nourishment of social relationships around mealtime.

This chapter addresses the following commonly asked questions about any eating and swallowing symptoms of a stroke:

- What is dysphagia?
- Why does my LO choke on coffee and water, eat so fast, drool, and have food trapped in their cheek?
- What is aspiration pneumonia?
- Why does my LO need a feeding tube? When can it be removed so that they can eat normally again?

WHAT IS DYSPHAGIA?

Dysphagia is a swallowing disorder that may occur because of weak or paralyzed muscles or because of a breakdown in the sequencing and timing of the complex swallow reflex.

Normally, there are three stages of swallowing: oral (in the mouth), pharyngeal (in the throat), and esophageal (from the esophagus to the stomach). Swallowing is actually a very complicated act that requires the coordination and precise timing of the 31 muscles involved. Each muscle must act at the right moment to allow food and liquid to successfully pass from the mouth to the stomach without any problems.

Swallowing problems may occur with different textures of food or liquid. They might occur in a single location or show multiple impairments with multiple locations in the mouth, pharynx, larynx, and/or esophagus. YouTube and Vimeo have many videos (such as this short one: *https://binged.it/2x0TfVa*) to help you visualize and understand both the anatomy and physiology of this complex reflex.

WHY DOES MY LO CHOKE ON WATER, EAT SO FAST, DROOL, AND HAVE FOOD TRAPPED IN THEIR CHEEK?

If your LO is coughing or choking when drinking or eating, it is a sign that something in the intricate process of swallowing is amiss. One of the many things a speech therapist (ST) or an occupational therapist (OT) will evaluate is your LO's ability to eat safely. A stroke may affect the muscles, coordination, and timing of the swallow, so that food or liquid could end up in the *trachea* (airway) instead of the *esophagus* (the tube that leads to the stomach). This is a critical issue because of the risk of *aspiration pneumonia*, a type of lung infection caused by oral bacteria, food, or vomit entering the lungs.

We've all had the experience of something "going down the wrong pipe," and our healthy bodies naturally cough as protection to clear our airways. Sometimes survivors lose this protective cough reflex, so instead of coughing and protecting their lungs, they have what's called *silent aspiration*. This "silent aspiration" puts them at *high risk* for developing aspiration pneumonia, which is a devastating infection that can be fatal.

A stroke survivor may have weakness, paralysis, or discoordination of the many oral muscles including the tongue, cheeks, and soft palate.

The tongue may be weak or paralyzed on one side, making them unable to adequately chew and form their food into a ball (or *bolus*) and move it around in their mouths. Next, the timing has to be just right for the swallow phase. Things can go wrong at many levels in the throat (the pharynx and larynx). Food can become trapped in various parts of the pharynx before it ultimately goes to either the windpipe or the stomach. These two pipes are like a forked highway, and the food has the opportunity to go down either one.

Therapists will perform bedside swallow evaluations to determine if a more comprehensive radiographic test is necessary to identify what textures and/or modifications for eating might be needed. Various textures of food are assessed at both the bedside swallowing test as well as during a formal swallow exam called *videofluoroscopy* or the Modified Barium Swallow test.

Your LO will be assessed to see if they can tolerate different consistencies, such as:

- Thin liquids (water, coffee, juice, broth, Jell-O™)
- Thick liquids (milkshake consistency)
- Pureed foods
- Small, soft foods
- Mechanically chopped food (small, cut-up pieces)
- Regular diet

Eating fast, taking too large of a bite, and incomplete chewing are all part of impulsivity and diminished sensory feedback for a stroke survivor. These factors present a risk for choking, aspiration, or at the very least an uncomfortable social problem. Helpful strategies are listed below in the Essential Answers section.

When cheek and tongue muscles are weak as seen in *hemiparesis* (partial paralysis on one half of the body) or *hemiplegia* (total paralysis on half of the body), food may get trapped in the affected side pockets of the cheeks and/or gums. It's important to make sure food is removed from these areas for two critical reasons:

1. Pocketed food (food trapped between the cheek and gums) could accidentally be ingested into the lungs

when the person is asleep. This could lead to aspiration pneumonia.

2. Pocketed food may cause dental decay.

WHAT IS ASPIRATION PNEUMONIA?

Aspiration pneumonia is a lung infection that occurs when food, saliva, liquids, or vomit is breathed into the lungs or into the airways leading to the lungs instead of being swallowed into the esophagus and stomach. This infection can lead to fatal consequences if not treated.

If you see any of the following signs of aspiration pneumonia, contact your doctor or nursing team immediately.

- Sudden, spiked fever
- Changes in the color of secretions (e.g., pus, mucus) from clear or white to yellow, green, and/or brown
- Blue lips
- Wet-sounding voice
- Wheezing
- Lethargy

A word about dental care in the hospital and at home. This *necessary* hygiene habit is routinely ignored in the hospital, especially if a LO isn't eating food orally and only receives nutrition through a feeding tube. It's critical to continue dental care, even if no oral food is taken for several reasons:

- Oral bacteria in the saliva can lead to aspiration pneumonia because we swallow between 600 and 700 times a day even if we're not eating.
- Oral bacteria leads to gum disease.
- Oral bacteria leads to inflammation throughout the body and is linked to increased cardiovascular problems.
- Oral bacteria can lead to tooth abscess and infections that can be painful and/or life-threatening.

Quenching Thirst with Dysphagia; "I'm just so thirsty" is a serious and chronic complaint we hear from stroke survivors. It's also a quality-of-life issue, especially for those on diets restricting thin liquids like water. While thickened liquids are offered as replacements, thickened water is anything but appealing or refreshing. People avoid what's unpleasant. Avoiding water is a problem.

Water is your body's most important nutrient. It's involved in every bodily function and makes up 70 to 75% of your total body weight. Water helps you maintain body temperature, metabolize body fat, aid digestion, lubricate and cushion organs, transport nutrients, and flush toxins from your body.

When people don't drink enough liquid, they can suffer dehydration. It only takes 2% dehydration for a person to start showing some warning signs.

Dehydration is potentially a very serious problem, which can result in severe outcomes including urinary tract infections (UTI). UTIs can cause cognitive symptoms that mimic a stroke. People with UTIs may become confused and disoriented; speech may be slurred and incomprehensible. UTIs can even lead to seizures. All of these symptoms scream neurological crisis, so if they happen to your LO, it's critical that your doctor rule out a UTI. Speak up when you see a sudden change in your LO's mental status, and ask about a potential UTI before the rehab team does another brain scan.

Dehydration may also impair memory and cause increased confusion, lethargy, heart palpitations, dizziness, low blood pressure, reduced effectiveness of medications, toxicity, irritability, delirium, muscle cramps (especially in the calves), dry mucous membranes, constipation, and even acute renal failure.

Since our cells need water for every function they perform, how does one deal with the risk of dehydration and keep potential aspirators safe?

First, discuss concerns about hydration with your nursing team and speech therapist. Next, familiarize yourself with the Frazier Water Protocol, an evidence-based program developed by Kathy Panther, MS, CCC-SLP, inpatient rehabilitation director at the Frazier Rehab Institute in Louisville, Kentucky. In short, this "free water" protocol allows patients who are NPO (Latin: *nil per os*), meaning nothing by mouth, or on thickened liquids to have ice chips or water *between* meals when following specific guidelines.

The protocol is not appropriate for every patient. You must consult your doctor and speech pathologist regarding its use. A link to the Frazier Water Protocol is provided in the Appendix under the Dysphagia heading. Meticulous oral hygiene is a key component of this protocol because it prevents bacteria from entering the lungs.

If the water protocol is not permitted, discuss hydration alternatives, such as IV fluids or foods with higher water content like yogurt. Inquire about the kind of oral care not dependent on swallowing that your LO can use to refresh their mouth and improve breath.

WHY DOES MY LO NEED A FEEDING TUBE? WHEN CAN IT BE REMOVED SO THAT THEY CAN EAT NORMALLY AGAIN?

Feeding tubes are given to people who are either comatose, barely alert, and/or have demonstrated swallowing problems that cannot be resolved quickly or do not allow the patient to safely receive adequate nutrition by mouth. These tubes may be temporary depending on the progress the individual patient makes during recovery.

Nasogastric or NG tubes (from the nose to stomach) are usually the first step. These tubes are inserted for short- or medium-term nutritional support not to exceed six weeks. Not everyone tolerates this. Patients often wittingly or unwittingly yank them out, creating a challenge for getting sustenance. If it is unsafe for your LO to eat food orally because they have known impairments as seen on videofluoroscopy or are not alert enough and if your doctor believes these problems will exceed six weeks, they may recommend a PEG feeding tube. PEG (percutaneous endoscopic gastrostomy) tubes require a minor surgical procedure wherein a feeding tube is inserted directly into the stomach through the skin.

Although PEG tubes reduce the chance of aspiration pneumonia, people can still aspirate on non-oral feedings. It's critical to make sure your LO remains in an upright position for any tube feeding to lessen the risk of reflux, regurgitation, and aspiration. PEG tubes also require specific care to maintain hygiene and lower the risk of infection at the skin site.

WHOSE TUBE IS IT, ANYWAY? A HOSPITAL TIP

Before your LO is discharged from the hospital, you *must* find out the name and phone number of the doctor who inserted their feeding tube and *who will be the one to remove it.* A patient discharged with a feeding tube is likely to fall through the cracks of care because of a "not my tube, not my responsibility" feeling among medical professionals who haven't inserted it. I've seen people with feeding tubes dangling from their bellies four months after they've resumed regular eating because no one wanted to be responsible for removing the tube.

After hospitalization, most medical care continues with your primary care doctors and not the hospital staff. Before a tube is removed, additional testing and/or videofluoroscopy may be needed to determine your LO's readiness to resume oral feedings. Obtain confirmation of *who* will remove the tube when the patient is discharged home. Do not accept the answer: "Your primary care doctor," as it is not correct. **Get the name and number of the person who inserted the tube and plan to follow up with that doctor.**

ESSENTIAL ANSWERS: What Makes It Better

- Correct positioning for eating is critical. Always make sure your LO is sitting bolt upright during the meal and for half an hour afterwards—including PEG tube feedings.
- Limit distractions during meals and avoid visitors who want to talk while your LO is eating.

- Give verbal and visual mirror feedback for wiping your LO's mouth. Because of decreased sensation, they may not feel that they have food on their face.

- Decrease "food shoveling" by giving the person a teaspoon versus a tablespoon.

- Remove visual distractions from the tray—have only the plate and silverware necessary.

- Make the meal attractive even if it's pureed food. (See the Appendix under Eating, Puree Food Molds.)

- Offer small portion sizes first. Give more food as requested. Too much food on a plate can psychologically turn off a person who has difficulty eating.

- If PEG tube feedings are given, learn to monitor the skin site where the tube is inserted. Always confirm that the name on the feeding bag matches your LO's name.

- Practice daily oral hygiene whether it is toothbrushing or oral swabbing, even if your LO is in ICU and has a feeding tube. Provide whatever assistance is needed. Hospitals provide sponge swabs, but if your LO can use an actual toothbrush, it's better. Floss. Many varieties of one-handed flossers are available and easily found at your local drugstore or even at the supermarket.

- Even if a person doesn't have teeth, oral care is necessary to reduce the amount of bacteria in saliva to prevent aspiration pneumonia.

- Learn the symptoms of aspiration pneumonia and contact nursing staff immediately if any appear.

- See the Appendix for resources under the Dysphagia header.

- Get in writing the name and phone number of the doctor who inserted the PEG tube and who will be responsible for its removal when your LO is discharged from the hospital.

ANSWERING YOUR MOST PRESSING
"WHY" QUESTIONS ABOUT
WALKING/
MOBILITY (C)

9
CHAPTER

> My doctor told me I would never walk again.
> My mother told me I would. I believed my mother.
> **~ Wilma Rudolph ~**
> *Olympic gold medalist and polio survivor*

Walking and mobility are the most basic and most desired skills of independence. For stroke survivors, impaired mobility can be psychologically distressing and frustrating, especially if your LO was very active before their stroke. In addition, long-term decreased mobility can impact many other physical factors including weight gain, fluid retention, skin sensitivity, pressure sores, and constipation.

So where is the hope? Remember neuroplasticity, the brain's spectacular capacity to create new pathways to rewire itself? Neuroplasticity is activated through repetition. Stroke survivors *can and do* recover the ability to walk independently when they are committed to consistent practice.

QUESTIONS ABOUT MOBILITY

- When will my LO walk again?
- When will my LO be able to use their arm and hand again?
- When will my LO be able to stay home alone?
- When can my LO drive?

WHEN WILL MY LO WALK AGAIN?

As mentioned earlier, walking is the most basic and most desired skill of independence, yet it is a complicated, integrated task that requires not just the legs, but the brain as well. So the annoying short answer is, *it depends.* Rehabilitative physical therapy may begin as soon as a person's overall condition is stabilized, often within 24 to 48 hours after the stroke. Initially a physical therapist may perform passive range of motion (PROM) exercises to maintain a paralyzed limb's muscle length and joint flexibility without the active participation of the survivor.

Muscle atrophy can begin very quickly, so preventative maintenance is easier than rebuilding lost muscle and flexibility. The next phase, active therapy, begins in bed. If a survivor is alert they are encouraged to change positions frequently and to begin a series of active range of motion exercises in bed. Actual walking requires a physical therapist's assessment. PTs will assess the survivor's sensation in the affected limb(s), their pain level, balance, coordination, blood pressure, reactivity, and *proprioception* (the brain's ability to know where the body is in space).

Physical therapists are nearly as eager as their patients to get them up and going, but safety is paramount. Falls are the biggest risk at this stage. Nothing undermines recovery more than an additional injury. Patients may progress from sitting up and moving with assistance between the bed and a chair to standing, bearing their own weight, and walking with or without assistance. Survivors using walkers and canes often ask therapists, "When will I walk again?" They ask this, *even while they're actually walking.* The desire to walk independently is so strong that walking with an assistive device doesn't feel like *real* walking.

It's critical to recognize the incremental steps of achieving a goal. *Walking is walking* regardless if it starts out with an assistive device. *That's a win!* It may not be your LO's *end goal,* but being able to *recognize and celebrate where they are for the moment* is an incremental step to knowing where they can be with continued practice.

Movement Recovery Based in Principles of Neuroplasticity

Two types of physical therapy you will *not* see in U.S. hospitals, but are worthy of your investigation are based on the principles of neuroplasticity. The Feldenkrais® Method is highly touted by Dr. Norman Doidge, psychiatrist, neuroplasticity expert, and the author of *The Brain's Way of Healing*. The Anat Baniel Method (ABM)® NeuroMovement® is an offshoot of Feldenkrais, as Baniel developed her method by expanding upon the principles of Feldenkrais.

The Feldenkrais Method was developed in the early 1950s, by Moshe Feldenkrais, a distinguished engineer, physicist, inventor, and martial arts expert. After suffering a crippling knee injury, Feldenkrais began to develop the protocols of his current renowned method, using his own body as his laboratory. By combining his insights from physics, motor development, biomechanics, psychology, and martial arts, he developed protocols to eliminate deeply embedded dysfunctional motor patterns. The Feldenkrais methods fall into what Dr. Doidge refers to as the final stage of neuroplastic healing. That is, the stage of *neurodifferentiation* when the brain is regulated and able to make fine distinctions.

Dr. Feldenkrais developed two teaching modalities: Awareness through Movement and Functional Integration. His work is built upon a fundamental principle of being able to distinguish and differentiate the most subtle of movements in order to repattern them because, as Feldenkrais said, "No part of the body can be moved without all the others being affected." To learn more about this modality and to find local practitioners, use this link: *www.feldenkrais.com/practitioner-search/*.

According to Dr. Jill Bolte Taylor, the neuroscientist who suffered a serious brain hemorrhage and chronicled both her stroke and her recovery in her book, *My Stroke of Insight*, the Anat Baniel Method® mimics what she intuitively did herself to recover her ability to walk. Although Dr. Taylor doesn't typically endorse products or services, she herself enrolled in the practitioner training of the Anat Baniel Method* and has remarked that she is a "big fan of this method" because it's consistent with the principles of neuroplasticity and neurological recovery.

Anat Baniel's Method NeuroMovement is significantly different from traditional physical therapy both conceptually and in practice.

The Baniel Method shifts the focus from the mechanical approach of trying to fix the body to focusing on the master organizer and controller of the body, the *brain*. The Anat Baniel Method utilizes Nine Essentials to wake up the brain and provide it with the conditions to generate new information and to differentiate and integrate new neural patterns. To learn more about her method, find practitioners, and obtain Baniel's free e-book, use this link: *https://fs234-21d9a3.pages.infusionsoft.net/*.

See the Appendix for additional links about these two methods.

ESSENTIAL ANSWERS: What Makes It Better

- Consult with the PT to learn the level of support and assistance your LO needs. Don't overhelp to the point where you create dependence.

- Encourage your LO to move often and always with safety awareness.

- Encourage your LO to use their stroke-impaired limbs, even though and *especially* because it's awkward. Remember neuroplasticity—the Use It or Lose It principle? Newly awakening nerve cells are primed to connect and build new pathways, but only if stimulated by repetitive action and practice.

- Investigate the Feldenkrais Method and/or the Anat Baniel Method and find practitioners to teach your LO how to repattern movements for walking and mobility.

WHEN WILL MY LO BE ABLE TO USE THEIR ARM AND HAND AGAIN?

Sounds like a simple and reasonable question, but first it's helpful to understand the complexity of what happens when an arm is either fully paralyzed or weakened. Problems start with the shoulder. The shoulder blade (or *scapula*) and the upper arm bone (or *humerus*) come together to form the shoulder joint. This joint is shaped like a ball and socket. When a paralyzed arm hangs, the weight of it can cause the shoulder joint to partially dislocate or separate. This is called a *subluxation*. The shoulder droops and feels as if it's out of joint. Muscles, tendons, and ligaments can become overstretched and may cause pain with movement. These muscle problems can lead to a reduced range of motion.

Can a paralyzed arm recover function, and if so, how? Yes, a paralyzed arm may recover either partial or full function. Let's look at how through the work of Signe Brunnström, a Swedish American OT and PT. In the 1960s she developed the Brunnström Approach, a seven-stage process for restoring motor control, recognizing that spasticity and primitive motor movements were part of the normal recovery process.

First, according to this approach, a stroke causes muscles to weaken due to the lack of coordination between the brain and body. As a result abnormal patterns of muscle *synergies* occur. "Synergies" here means using bundled movements of multiple joints to accomplish something usually done by one joint. For example, a person might use their elbow, shoulder, and hand as a unit to accomplish the simple act of bending just their hand. The Brunnström Approach teaches people how to use these abnormal synergy patterns to their advantage.

Not all therapists agree with this approach. In fact, some believe it's best to inhibit these abnormal patterns early, lest they become habitual. But there's also a great deal of research and evidence with Constraint-Induced Therapy suggesting that *any* movement is good movement and with enough "massed practice" (practicing a movement many hours a day for a period of several weeks), the synergistic movements will begin to disappear in favor of normal patterns.

Constraint-Induced Therapy *reStrains* (not retrains) the functioning arm or hand by way of a mitt, permitting only the stroke-affected arm to move. It focuses on "massed practice"— meaning lots of repetition, concentrating an extraordinary amount of exercise in a couple of weeks. CIT is the most researched and clinically proven stroke recovery option. A person must have some tone and movement present to use this approach. For more information see the Appendix under Resources for OT and PT.

Brunnström Seven Stages of Recovery

Stage 1: Flaccidity.

A complete lack of voluntary movement, commonly referred to as paralysis.

Stage 2: Spasticity.

Muscles begin to make small, spastic, and abnormal movements during this stage. Even though these movements are mostly involuntary, they can be a promising sign. Minimal voluntary movements might or might not be present in Stage 2.

Stage 3: Increased Spasticity.

Spasticity is a feeling of unusually stiff, tight, or pulled muscles that may interfere with movement or cause pain. It is caused by damage to the nerve pathways within the brain or spinal cord that controls muscle movement. The lack of ability to restrict the brain's motor neurons causes muscles to contract too often. Spasticity during this phase reaches its peak. While this is very uncomfortable, alarming, and seems counterintuitive as a sign of progress, it is a vital component of recovery.

During Stage 3, synergy patterns begin to emerge. Begin to look for and expect minimal voluntary movements. A survivor may begin to *initiate* movement in the muscle, but not be able to *control* it (yet).

People experiencing severe spasticity are typically more limited in their ability to exercise independently, but it's critical that your LO maintain range of motion and do daily exercises. Therapeutic assistance from an OT or a caregiver trained in passive range of motion (PROM) exercises is important.

Stage 4: Decreased Spasticity.

During this stage, spastic muscle movement begins to decline. As people begin to regain control in their extremities and demonstrate limited ability to move normally, the focus of therapy shifts to strengthening and improving muscle control. Stretching and ROM exercises are still important in this stage.

Therapists use *active assisted range of motion exercises* (AAROM) to help the survivor who has some ability to move but still needs help to practice the exercises or complete the movements. A therapist may help guide a movement with their own body (holding the limb, for example) or through the use of bands and other exercise equipment. See the Appendix for more information on occupational therapy aids and equipment.

Active ROM (AROM) exercises begin once a person has regained some muscle control and can perform some exercises without assistance. Exercises may involve moving a limb along its full range of motion, like bending an elbow or rotating a wrist. AROM exercises increase flexibility, muscle strength, and endurance. Range of motion exercises should be practiced equally on both the affected and unaffected sides of the body. It's best to consult with an OT to customize a plan, demonstrate specific exercises, and recommend appropriate aids and equipment.

Stage 5: Complex Movement Combinations.

In Stage 5, declining spasticity allows for more coordinated muscle patterns to emerge. You will see your LO making more controlled and deliberate movements in affected limbs. Isolated joint movements might also be possible. Abnormal movements also start to decline dramatically during Stage 5, but some may still be present.

All voluntary movements start within the brain. Motor signals are initiated by thought and must involve sensory stimuli. Incorporating visual, auditory, and kinesthetic cues in thinking about movement aids the brain's ability to send a motor signal to muscles, ligaments, and joints.

A therapist working on getting someone to open and close their hand might ask them to imagine that they are a giant scooping up and squashing little monsters till they feel them explode. Okay, it's a bit graphic, but the brain needs to see it, hear it, and feel it to make it move. When thoughts are robust they activate more neurons, and as stated before, it's the connections among neurons firing together that creates new neural pathways. Active thinking transforms a weak open/close hand gesture into a more dynamic and functional movement. *Think:* Go big or Go home.

Stage 6: Spasticity Disappears.

Huge progress at this stage: spasticity in muscle movement disappears completely. A person is able to move individual joints, and their synergy patterns become much more coordinated. Motor control is almost fully restored, and one can coordinate complex reaching movements in the affected extremities. Abnormal or spastic movements have ceased, and a full recovery may be on the horizon.

Stage 7: Normal Function Returns.

The final stage of the Brunnström Approach is when a survivor regains full function in the areas affected by the stroke. They are now able to move their arms and hands in a controlled manner.

The big question is, "How long does it take, and does everyone achieve full recovery?"

How long it takes depends once again on many factors: the level of mobility impairment, the frequency and intensity of stimulation and exercise, whether any medical conditions coexist, and the survivor's determination and motivation to heal. That said, recovery may take anywhere from several weeks to several months to several years, and may even be a lifelong process. Consult with your doctor and OT or PT regarding the management of spasticity and the maintenance of ongoing exercises and stretching.

Does everyone recover function? Regrettably no. Some may begin recovery but get stuck in the spastic stage wherein muscle tightness causes the elbow to be bent for many hours a day for days on end. The result is that the arm pulls up in a position similar to a chicken wing. If the muscles and soft tissue permanently shorten, it will become impossible to straighten the elbow. This fixed position is known as a *contracture*. The joint is literally immovable even if someone else tries to passively range it. The only way to avoid contractures is with stretching and ROM exercises. Peter G. Levine's book, *Stronger After Stroke,* offers comprehensive information on spasticity control and elimination. See Suggested Readings in the back of the book.

ESSENTIAL ANSWERS: What Makes It Better

- Stretching and range of motion (ROM) exercises.
- Strength training for hand grip and building muscle.
- Constraint-Induced Movement Therapy: *Restraining* the functioning hand to allow the affected one to do as much work as possible.
- Tone management techniques include: (use of an air splint, weight bearing activities, the prolonged stretch of a muscle group, and a type of massage called myofascial release).
- Sensory stimulation to improve motor planning and proprioceptive awareness of what muscle groups to activate.
- Electrical stimulation to stimulate muscle contraction, reduce pain and spasticity.
- Mirror therapy: A mirror is placed between the affected limb and the functioning limb. The survivor sees only the functioning limb in the mirror. As movements are made with the healthy limb, the survivor simultaneously tries to move the affected limb. This optical illusion tricks the

brain into perceiving the affected limb is moving normally and often helps the brain rewire itself to improve mobility. Use this link to learn more and find exercises to try at home *www.flintrehab.com/2018/mirror-therapy-stroke/*. See Appendix under OT resources for a link to a video showing how the exercises are performed.

- Fine motor skill practice: Trace designs with a pen, use a pegboard, pick up small beans and transfer to cup, shuffle cards. Practice, practice, practice.
- Consult your doctor to determine if oral medication for spasticity can help. Discuss the risks and benefits of medicine as they may cause drowsiness and weakness.
- Consult your doctor about the use of botulinum and/ or phenol injections to help with spasticity. (Injection effectiveness can last from three to six months.)
- Consult with your doctor to discuss intrathecal baclofen, a small surgically implanted pump that administers a muscle relaxant to the spinal fluid. This is used for severe spasticity or when someone has not done well on oral meds.
- Investigate neuroplastic therapeutic modalities for recovering motor abilities: The Feldenkrais Method and the Anat Baniel Method.

WHEN WILL MY LO BE ABLE TO STAY HOME ALONE?

As a caregiver and perhaps the sole supporter of the family, it's important to know when you might go back to work or attend to the many details of your life that have been put on hold since your LO's stroke. The short answer is, *it depends*. Let's look at the three things needed for your LO to be safe at home alone.

- Physical mobility and stability
- Cognitive ability
- Household accessibility and safety features

A paralyzed person in a wheelchair with adequate communication skills, a good memory, intact judgement and problem-solving abilities can easily be independent. Cognitive skills include a person's judgement, impulsivity, reasoning, and problem-solving skills.

You and your LO should discuss their strengths, weaknesses, and potential needs before you leave them home alone. A survivor's self-awareness is a critical component of cognition as it determines their safety and ability to self-regulate.

Below is a list of the typical questions you should ask when determining your LO's level of safety, readiness, and anticipated needs for staying alone. The best way to determine readiness is a melding of opinions from the survivor and caregiver, along with professional observations and tests from the PT, OT, ST, and social worker.

- Is your home/dwelling accessible and safe? Are there clear pathways for a wheelchair or walker?
- Has your LO demonstrated competency and safety navigating the house independently or with whatever assistive device they are using?
- How is their balance? Their reaction time? Can they recover if they misstep?
- Are the bathrooms equipped with grab bars, raised toilet seats, and/or other necessary aids?
- Have slippery rugs been removed?
- Does your LO neglect their affected side and bump into things, making falls more likely?
- Has your LO practiced fall recovery? That is, can they get up from the floor if they fall?
- Can your LO safely and independently leave the house if there is an emergency?
- Can your LO communicate effectively?
- Can your LO call for help either by phone or using a Call Alert device?
- How are your LO's problem-solving skills? Can they assess home emergencies?
- How are your LO's reasoning skills? Would they invite strangers into the home or be at risk for talking to solicitors either at the door or on the phone?

- Does your LO have short-term memory problems? Will your LO be at risk if cooking?
- Does your LO have something to do that is stimulating and rewarding besides watch TV?
- What is your LO's emotional status? Depressed? Anxious? Impulsive?
- Will your LO's emotional status lead to dangerous outcomes? Impulsivity might lead to climbing on ladders, operating machinery, or trying to drive. Depression and anxiety might lead to overmedication with alcohol or other drugs.
- Is the house equipped with *functioning* smoke and carbon monoxide detectors?

Once you can answer these questions with confidence and your LO has the official "sign-off" from their team, you may leave them home alone for predetermined amounts of time.

WHEN CAN MY LO DRIVE?

Answering "When can your LO drive?" of course starts with *It depends.* Next to walking, driving is the single most yearned-for activity and often the most contentiously debated topic between caregivers and survivors. Driving is the ultimate hallmark of independence, but there is a lot at stake behind the wheel.

Driving is a very complex task requiring many skills. First one needs intact visual skills including good acuity, eye coordination, color vision, contrast sensitivity, the ability to see in low light at night, depth perception, and peripheral vision. Stroke survivors may have visual field cuts that prevent them from seeing halves or quarters of what's around them. You might see evidence of this when your LO constantly bumps into things on one side or completely ignores the food on one side of their plate. They may experience double vision or have depth perception difficulties. Typically a person is advised to wait approximately six months after a stroke before obtaining new corrective lenses because vision is in a constant state of flux during this period of recovery.

Not only is vision a concern while driving, but so are motor ability and cognitive function, including: memory, reasoning, problem-solving, judgement, impulsivity and emotional stability, and reaction time/processing speed.

In some states, doctors are legally responsible to notify the DMV if someone suffers a lapse of consciousness or has a seizure condition. In my experience, most often doctors don't report this. They assume the patient will act responsibly and safely and not undertake driving until they are capable.

Most physiatrists (rehab specialists) have a strict policy of waiting a minimum of six months before allowing a survivor to drive. Some rehab facilities offer driving simulators for use as both an assessment tool and for practice.

Getting a professional driving evaluation is the best way to ensure everyone's safety and confidence before your LO gets back behind the wheel. A doctor must provide a prescription for a survivor to have their driving skills tested by an OT. Driving assessments are typically not covered by insurance and cost approximately $400 to $600.

Driving assessments are not like DMV tests. OTs will assess both cognitive and motor skills in real-life behind-the-wheel conditions on local roads and highways in vehicles equipped with passenger-side brakes. OTs will also test pathfinding, memory, and the knowledge of road signs as well as how well one manages a variety of on-road challenges. At the conclusion of the test, the OT will write a report either confirming a survivor's readiness for driving or making suggestions about the areas they still need to work on.

If motor impairment is the only challenge, modifications can be made to enable survivors to get behind the wheel of their car. Adaptations might include hand controls, left-foot accelerators, lifts, and mobility seating. The cost of these modifications can vary greatly. See Appendix Resources under the category of Driving.

Randy was the owner of his software company. Before his stroke, if he wasn't working, he was trekking mountains or going on weekend bike trips into the wilderness. Initially frustrated by not being able to drive due to his vision and memory problems, Randy found a silver lining to his temporary situation. His healthy, 80-year-old father offered to provide him with transportation. During their drive time, Randy reconnected with his dad, laughing, reminiscing, and playing the word games they had played on car trips when he was a child. Randy realized the gift of spending time with his elderly father and how much he'd actually missed him. He also found playing those vocabulary games helped improve his memory.

A great many stroke survivors eventually return to driving. Patience, time, and persistence all help.

ESSENTIAL ANSWERS: What Makes It Better

- Getting an accurate assessment of driving skills.
- Learning about alternative transportation. (For a deeper dive, see Chapter 26: Driving & Working.)
- Being open to receiving help from family and friends.

ANSWERING YOUR MOST PRESSING
"WHY" QUESTIONS ABOUT
COGNITION/
MEMORY (C)

10
CHAPTER

Every man's memory is his private literature.
~ Aldous Huxley ~

Cognition is the ability to think and know. Cognition involves complex processes like attention, memory, reasoning, decision-making, problem-solving, and the subsets of *executive function*, which include planning, initiating, directing, and self-monitoring. When it comes to cognition and memory after stroke, some of the common questions caregivers and families ask are:

- Why does my LO forget information from one day to the next?
- Why does my LO get lost? Why can't they recognize where they are?
- Why doesn't my LO initiate anything?
- Why doesn't my LO trust us? Why do they think we are trying to control them?

WHY DOES MY LO FORGET INFORMATION FROM ONE DAY TO THE NEXT?

Short-term memory loss is a common occurrence with stroke. Families are confounded as to why their LO can remember things from 40 years ago, but can't remember what someone told them 5 minutes ago. Short-term memory is sometimes called working memory. It's brief and fleeting. It's similar to the memory of your computer when you're working on a document. Unless you hit save, that information will be lost. Working memory is only converted into long-term memory if there is enough attention and *collateral sensory information* (such as a visual, auditory, or tactile/kinesthetic) to literally hit the SAVE button and transport and consolidate the information into long-term memory.

Many factors interfere with memory. Decreased or absent attention is the first and foremost factor. Pain, fatigue, medications, alcohol and drugs, and overstimulation all interfere with attention and therefore impact memory. If your LO is in pain, they won't be able to focus on higher-level activities like challenging conversations or strenuous physical tasks.

ESSENTIAL ANSWERS: What Makes It Better

- If pain is the issue, have your LO rate the severity on a scale from one to five. If their pain is higher than a three, discuss possible solutions with your doctor. Also discuss any medications you may suspect are interfering with your LO's memory. Painkillers are the most likely culprits. Medication is always about balancing the risks and the benefits, and that decision is best made with your LO and doctor. Know that you may have to experiment before you get it right.
- Adequate rest is critical to allowing long-term memories to consolidate.
- Keep simple journals to help your LO become and stay oriented by invoking new visual, auditory, and/or tactile memories.

> ### Journal Entry Example:
>
> Sunday, Feb. 11, 2018. 9:00 am.
>
> Fred visited with coffee and muffins from Martha's Bakery. He joked about his new boss.

This entry includes sensory details from all three modalities:

Visual: The image of Fred and the muffins.

Auditory: The sound of joking and laughing.

Tactile/Kinesthetic: How it feels, smells, and tastes to eat fresh muffins.

- Avoid *testing* memory. Instead use the journal as a springboard for conversation that *reinforces* and *stabilizes* your LO's memory. Prime your LO with the memory and *then* discuss it: "Remember, yesterday Fred came with muffins and coffee and joked about his boss. What did you think of that?" Priming them with the actual memory and using the word "Remember" subtly gives the brain direction and focus while respecting and preserving your LO's dignity. You are not asking *if* they remember, you are directing the brain *to remember*. Make sure you modulate your tone so the word "Remember" sounds like a *directive*, not a question, which would have a rising inflection. However, if the word "remember" triggers unwanted responses (e.g., "NO, STOP ASKING ME IF I REMEMBER!"), avoid using it.

- Record short video visits or take photos you can discuss throughout the day: "Look at this. Remember when Rita came...."

- Provide a large whiteboard calendar and have your LO mark the days off. Put special events on the calendar— especially a projected discharge date and other meaningful activities and events.

- Greet your LO every day with, "Hi, it's _____ (name the day and date), let's see what's on your schedule for today."

- If your LO can write, have them keep a journal. Record important or memorable events each day.

- Use this book's companion journal, *Hope After Stroke: My Recovery Journal,* to find easy and comprehensive memory cues and notes for recording progress.

- If your LO can speak but not write, have them dictate three events that happened that day. Write them down and ask your LO to read it.

WHY DOES MY LO GET LOST? WHY CAN'T THEY RECOGNIZE WHERE THEY ARE?

Strokes occurring on the right side of the brain can be tricky for doctors who spend a brief amount of time talking to the survivors. This is because right brain strokes often cause disorientation in place and time. Often speech and language are unimpaired and the patient seems very reasonable, insightful, and competent. Even so, survivors may get lost or have difficulty navigating even in familiar areas. These impairments tend to surface once a person is home. Caregivers are usually the first to notice.

> Fred was a renowned pharmacist specializing in the unique field of pharmacokinetics. Physicians from around the country consulted him to know what medications and dosages to use with their highest-risk and most medically complicated patients. Then, Fred suffered a right brain stroke. I first met him at his home shortly after his hospitalization. His speech and language were perfectly intact.
>
> "I want you to tell me the truth," he said.
>
> "What's the truth you want?" I asked.
>
> "Everyone tells me I'm *home* and I must admit this place is decorated *very similarly*, but I know I am *not* home."
>
> No amount of factual proof convinced him. Eventually he learned to accept the pleasant, "similarly decorated" place, even though he *knew* it wasn't his home. It took his family some time to accept this change in their LO.

ESSENTIAL ANSWERS: What Makes It Better

- Not trying to prove you are right and they are wrong.
- Keeping them safe while honoring their dignity.

- Repetition of paths to and from familiar locations with them guiding the way—allow for errors and observe problem-solving skills used.
- Increase independence by using phone apps for walking navigation.

WHY DOESN'T MY LO INITIATE ANYTHING?

Apathetic behavior can occur after a stroke when an intracerebral hemorrhage has damaged the right hemisphere. Your LO may just sit and stare. This apathy may be mistaken for depression, but it may be a condition called *abulia* (ay-BOOL-ee-ya). Abulia is clinically distinct from depression. People with abulia typically do not exhibit signs of sadness or negative thoughts. Abulia shows up as a lack of concern about one's condition or the world around them. In extreme cases a person may become mute even though they are able to speak. Your doctor must help differentiate between the disorders as the treatments are very different.

ESSENTIAL ANSWERS: What Makes It Better

- Medical evaluation with appropriate medication.
- Provide your LO with the choice between two or three activities, such as what to do or where to go, but make it clear that they will choose something. Get them to stand and initiate movement as a first step.

WHY DOESN'T MY LO TRUST US? WHY DO THEY THINK WE ARE TRYING TO CONTROL THEM?

This distrust, even to the level of seeming paranoia, is a common characteristic of a person who's had damage to the right hemisphere of their brain. They often feel people are lying to them or withholding information. At the extreme, survivors may accuse their family members of holding them prisoner and preventing them from driving and other previous acts of independence.

Once again, what's most confusing for family, caregivers, and even doctors, who typically have short conversations with these survivors, is that they don't *sound* like they have a brain injury. They sound perfectly sensible. Their speech is clear and articulate; their voice, rhythm, and pacing sound normal. They seem to be coherent, reasonable, and make sense, but those who suffer right hemisphere brain damage often have severe memory, reasoning, sensory, and judgement problems. They perceive they are far more capable than they are, especially when it comes to driving. They may become disoriented to place and time, lose their way, and suffer sensory disturbances.

Your LO's lack of reasoning, insight, and self-monitoring may make it unsafe for them to be left alone because their impaired memory and judgement present dangers, especially if they decide to cook, climb on a ladder, drive, or use a chainsaw to trim the trees. See Chapter 9: Answering Your Most Pressing "Why" Questions about Walking/Mobility to assess how you can know if a LO can be left home alone.

ESSENTIAL ANSWERS: What Makes It Better

- Provide small opportunities for independence. In the hospital, encourage ambulatory survivors (even those in wheelchairs who can manage independently) to get to the therapy room independently for their appointments.
- At home, try an outing to a small store where a caregiver stands outside by the exit. Make sure there is only one exit. Agree to meet at a specific location and time. Make certain your LO has a phone, so you can call in case they don't arrive at the designated location.
- When driving, ask your LO to give you verbal directions to familiar places, such as the grocery store, gas station, or post office.
- Occasionally take a wrong turn and see if they recognize it's wrong. If so, see if they can guide you to a new path or return to the original path.

- Discuss driving with your doctor and LO. See Chapter 26: Driving & Working for more information.
- Car keys may have to be temporarily locked away. Make sure other family members understand the severity of the safety issue. Do not allow friends or family members to be talked into handing over car keys in order to do the LO a *favor.*

SOCIAL/ EMOTIONAL BEHAVIORS (C)

11
CHAPTER

What we achieve inwardly will change our outer reality.
~ Plutarch ~

After a stroke, people commonly experience social, emotional, and behavioral changes. The physical effects of stroke are *visible* and that which we see, in some ways, is more easily understood. It is the personality and emotional changes that may be more puzzling and troubling for both the survivor and caregiver. These *invisible* effects of brain damage affect more than a third of stroke survivors.

As such, you'll likely want to know:

- Why is my LO so depressed and/or angry? Why do they cry so easily?
- Why is my LO so anxious and easily agitated?
- Why is my LO so impulsive?
- Why does my LO self-isolate and want to leave a place as soon as we get there?

WHY IS MY LO SO DEPRESSED AND/OR ANGRY? WHY DO THEY CRY SO EASILY?

Imagine the fear and confusion of waking up in a hospital and realizing your limbs are paralyzed, that half of your body is useless. You can't roll over or sit up. You can't walk. (By the way many survivors are in such a deep state of denial, they don't believe they're paralyzed, and incur even greater injuries from a fall as they attempt to walk.)

People you don't know touch and move you, poke and prod you, and awaken you by sticking a needle in your arm. Your dignity and privacy are gone, you can't even use the bathroom by yourself. Now imagine trying to talk, your lips and tongue thick and uncoordinated and your words nonexistent. They're stuck in your head, but nothing comes out. Language has vanished. Or maybe you're talking up a blue streak, but the "idiots" around you shove whiteboards and markers at you because they can't understand you. Sensory information bombards you, keeping you up at all hours of the day and night. Flashing lights, beeping noises, and a cacophony of incomprehensible "word" sounds assault your senses. You want to bury your head in the covers and make this stop. This is your living nightmare.

As the survivor comes to terms with the effects of their stroke, the emotions of frustration, anger, sadness, and grief are considered "normal," but normal emotions aren't the same as *desired* ones. These radical life changes are hard on everyone, not just the survivor. Crying and emotional fragility are common for even the formerly stoic. First, there are *justifiable* reasons for these increased negative emotions. Second, there may be actual damage to the brain that is causing personality changes like disinhibition, increased agitation, and depression. Third, after a major life event people are naturally more emotionally vulnerable. When one is faced with their own mortality and the reality of how fragile life is, the facade of having everything under control may crumble. Previously controlled and repressed emotions surface more readily. For a deeper dive into depression and anxiety related to stroke, see Chapter 18 "Tapping" Down Anxiety, Pain, & Overwhelm.

A stroke has a way of turning up the volume on emotions. Whatever your LO's *premorbid* (before stroke) behavior was like, it will likely be exaggerated after they've had a stroke. If they were short-tempered, anxious, or depressed before the stroke, you will likely see a worsening of those behaviors, at least in the short term. An appropriate level of emotional expression, even if it's sadness, is expected and shouldn't be confused with another disorder called *pseudobulbar affect* (PBA), which is caused by frontal lobe damage.

PBA is a secondary neurologic condition that causes excessive, sudden, unpredictable, *inappropriate* or uncontrollable laughing or crying that doesn't match how one feels. Other emotional outbursts like agitation, impulsivity, and disinhibition may also be the result of frontal lobe damage and are not considered within the normal expected range of emotions. If you're unsure which disorder your LO is experiencing, ask your doctor to test for confirmation.

WHY IS MY LO SO ANXIOUS AND EASILY AGITATED?

If your LO was a smoker, alcoholic or heavy drinker, user of recreational drugs, opioids, or other mood-altering substances, let the doctor know. In addition to dealing with their obvious medical and neurological issues, they are likely in withdrawal. It's possible a LO may become physically aggressive and abusive, especially if there is a history of alcoholism or drug abuse or if your LO was actively drinking or using narcotics or other illegal drugs directly before their stroke.

If your LO's anger, depression, anxiety, and inappropriate emotion are excessive, persistent, and interfering with life–in other words, not episodic and likely related to frustration–talk to your doctor and/or a psychiatrist to see if medication is a viable solution.

It's always a good idea to experiment with common-sense solutions before resorting to medication to see if your LO's mood, affect, and behavior improve. These common sense approaches include: adequate rest, increased hydration, regulated meals, optimized communication, and appropriate levels of stimulation while preventing overstimulation. Medication may or may not be the "magic pill." For some people, certain medications can radically improve mood and behavior, while for others, those same medications actually worsen conditions. Report ongoing changes as medications are used. Expect to wait two or more weeks to notice improvements as antidepressants take time to work.

You must recognize when a LO's behavior is unmanageable and dangerous. Do not allow a sense of duty or embarrassment to put you or your family at risk. You must seek the help of a social worker, doctor, and/or counselor to determine how best to manage their behavior and to potentially help find alternative living arrangements that keep you and other family members safe. It is best to proactively address physical aggression with your medical providers rather than resorting to calling law enforcement. However, if you do not seek these services and aggression escalates to the point that you believe your physical safety is threatened, you may need to contact the police. **Make certain to lock away any firearms or weapons and strictly prohibit access to them.** A person with a brain injury and known agitation should not have access to guns or weapons, no matter what.

WHY IS MY LO SO IMPULSIVE?

Damage to the frontal lobe or to the right side of the brain often results in impulsivity. Safety is the biggest concern for people with this type of injury and behavior. Your LO's inability to predict consequences, combined with poor self-awareness and judgement, make them prone to accidents, especially if they have motor or balance impairments. These are the folks who, when left alone at home, may decide to use ladders, clean the roof, trim the trees, or engage in otherwise dangerous activities that exceed their physical and cognitive limits.

Falls are the greatest and most likely risk in this situation. Falls typically occur either on the way to the bathroom or in it because there is usually urgency around relieving one's self. Bathrooms are the most dangerous place because of their hard and slippery surfaces. Accidents may happen when a survivor is impulsive in making transitions to and from the shower and toilet. While no one can predict how long impulsive behavior will last, in many cases, it will subside or lessen with time and recovery. The goal is to optimize safety while encouraging increasing independence. See Chapter 9: Answering Your Most Pressing "Why" Questions about Walking/Mobility for an assessment tool to help determine when a LO may safely stay home alone.

ESSENTIAL ANSWERS: What Makes It Better

- Report any previous history of drug use, smoking, or alcoholism to help manage possible withdrawal symptoms.
- Manage stress and fatigue. Impulsivity worsens under both conditions. Watch for trigger signs. It's easier to avert the problem than to manage it.
- Catch them doing something well. "Your balance really improves when you take a second to stand before walking."
- Ask questions gently: "What did the PT say would make you safer on walks?"
- Consult with your physician or social worker if your LO's behavior is aggressive and dangerous.
- Lock away firearms and do not let an impulsive and agitated person have access to any weapons.
- Use common sense approaches to managing frustration and anxiety such as adequate rest, regulated meals, hydration and low level stimulation along with or in place of medication for mood and affect.

WHY DOES MY LO SELF-ISOLATE AND WANT TO LEAVE A PLACE AS SOON AS WE GET THERE?

Overstimulation may be the most simple explanation. There may be just too much information bombarding the brain. Imagine your worst headache and then imagine going to a noisy place in a foreign country where you don't speak the language. There are bright lights and fast-moving conversations where people ask you questions and demand fast answers. The attentional demands exceed your LO's ability, so isolation becomes a means of shutting down the assaultive experience that's just too uncomfortable.

Anxiety may also account for a survivor's desire to withdraw from or avoid situations as 20% of stroke survivors experience some type of anxiety right after a stroke.

ESSENTIAL ANSWERS: What Makes It Better

- Consult a mental healthcare professional such as a doctor, social worker, or psychologist who specializes in stroke-related injuries to explore if medications or therapy are needed to manage and improve your LO's depressive or anxious symptoms.
- Engage in support groups for both the caregiver and the survivor.
- Optimize safety for those with impulsive behavior. Gradually encourage independence.
- Experiment with common-sense solutions for mood swings, depression, and anxiety: adequate rest, increased hydration, regulated meals, appropriate levels of stimulation, optimized communication.
- Medication may or may not be the "magic pill." Report ongoing changes (both positive and negative) as medications are used. Expect to wait two or more weeks to notice improvements as antidepressants take time to work.
- See Chapter 18: "Tapping" Down Anxiety, Pain, & Overwhelm for a non-medicinal self-help tool.
- Always consult your doctor before using natural mood enhancers or cannabinoid products.

DRESSING FOR SUCCESS (C&S)

*You cannot climb the ladder of success
dressed in the costume of failure.*
~ Zig Ziglar ~

Some people think of recovery as a final destination. They might say, "When I recover, I'll get my life back" or "When I recover, I'll be happy." Recovery, however, is not a final destination; recovery is a daily journey.

When I enter a patient's hospital room or visit them at home and they're dressed, I know they're in a recovery mindset. Survivors who want to be well get up and get dressed. Survivors who are sick or who view themselves as sick are slower to start. There are medical factors, of course, that can complicate readiness, like an underlying disease process, severe pain, poor adjustment to medication, and wildly fluctuating blood pressure or sugar levels. However, assuming a person is medically stable and in the subacute phase of recovery, this is prime time for suiting up and showing up.

Sometimes a survivor will talk about their prior life saying, "Before I got sick…" Since I'm a stickler for language and know how our words shape our reality, not just describe it (as you learned in Chapter 5), I gently correct them. "You mean *before you had a stroke,*" I say.

Survivors are not "sick." A stroke is not an *illness,* it is the result of an underlying condition. A stroke is an event and an injury. It's true, a survivor may feel terrible and connect that feeling to the familiar label of being sick. It's also true that the underlying disease process, such as cardiovascular disease, also needs attention as part of the healing process. That said, even when one feels awful, anything that happens *after* the event (assuming there are no further medical complications) is part of the process of healing.

The importance of this *simple* mental shift from being *sick* to being in *recovery* is enormous.

> If you *think* you are healing you take entirely different steps. When you *believe* you will get and be better, your determination increases. You begin to look for and celebrate evidence of progress.
> **Yes, *thinking* you will be better is the single most important step to *becoming* and *being* better.**

Thoughts control everything, and science backs this up.

Injured Olympic athletes who can't physically train spend hours thinking, visualizing, and *feeling* what it's like to run their 100-meter dash or land a triple axel. This active engagement of their neurology keeps them primed to return to their sport.

Imagery, which includes all the senses, not just vision, is also used in the healing process. The Olympic freestyle aerialist skier Emily Cook used it to see and feel her bones heal as she worked through a two-year recovery after a ski crash left her with broken bones in both feet.

Of course, after they began thinking positively, these athletes eventually mended enough to suit up and work with their own rehab team of physical therapists to get back in the game. However, the thing that kept them going, and the thing that makes them stars, is their positive thought process, their magnification of the good. You can bring this mindset into your occupational, physical, and speech therapy sessions, too. All progress begins with a thought.

Science has long proven that our minds can change our bodies, but we're now learning that our bodies can change our brain chemistry. Dr. Amy Cuddy, a social psychologist and associate professor at the Harvard Business School, researched that very question: *Can your body fake it till your mind makes it?*

She studied whether simply changing one's body posture could affect a measurable change in the hormones associated with *dominance* (testosterone) and *stress* (cortisol). Turns out it did. Cuddy demonstrated that a powerful body pose (outstretched arms and legs to make the body bigger) assumed for only two minutes significantly raised testosterone levels, whereas striking a lower-power pose (closed in and smaller) increased cortisol. In other words, two minutes of assuming a specific body posture triggered hormones that shaped the brain to be either assertive, confident, and comfortable or stress-reactive and shut-down.

So, why is "faking it till you make it," or as I like to say, "acting as if," important to stroke survivors?

Meet Amber.

> Amber slept in her clothes for days on end. She said it was "just easier" as she pointed to her limp right arm. She cried often and talked about her fear of what was going to happen to her. I visited her in her home and noticed the shelves and mantles lined with framed photos of a statuesque and beautifully dressed woman wearing bright red lipstick, beaming a megawatt smile.
>
> "Amber," I said, "you gotta at least put on your lips, girlfriend." She rummaged through the purse at the foot of her bed and took out a tube of lipstick. With weak, uncoordinated, and shaky fingers, she dabbed it on her lips, while also getting it on her nose and chin. At first she seemed more discouraged, but then we both burst into laughter at the rocky start. There it was, Amber's megawatt, triumphant smile. Fueled with new confidence, her body opened up. She sat taller.
>
> When the OT brought out the tiny beans and cup, a previously loathed fine motor skills activity, Amber tackled it with the enthusiasm of a child operating a robotic claw in hopes of grasping a stuffed toy. This was now a game, and the more Amber persisted, the more capable her fingers became. Amber picked up one tiny bean after the next, chuckling at the sound of each kerplunk as it landed in the cup. The next time I visited Amber she was dressed in snazzy sweats, sparkly sneakers, and her lips glistened in candy apple red.

> **SUIT UP, SHOW UP, START UP,
> and STAY CONSISTENT**
>
> *Act as if you are who you want to be because
> every day you are becoming more of who you are.*

We automatically feel better, more dignified, more whole and intact when our teeth are brushed, our face is washed, and we're dressed to meet and work with others. If you need assistance with this, see the Appendix resources under Rehab-Ready Clothes especially for hemiplegics (those with one-sided paralysis).

When we feel confident, others see and think it, too, and when others see us making progress, they reinforce our efforts and their energy amplifies this message: I AM GETTING BETTER EACH AND EVERY DAY.

Each success must be acknowledged and celebrated. Healing and recovery are about seeing the tiny, incremental changes. Use a magnifying glass to look for and magnify the progress.

WHAT DO YOU LOOK FOR?

If you look for progress, you will see it. That's not to say you should ignore what's wrong. No, you must see things as they are, not better and not worse. If you objectively see what is working and what still needs work, you will continue to grow.

It's much like working in a garden. You can look at all the weeds and say, "This garden is a mess and not worth saving." Or you can say, "There are weeds here, but there's also fertile soil. I can remove the weeds and tend to the fertile soil. In time, I know flowers will bloom."

So, what does progress look like in the hospital?

- Your LO sat up for increasing periods of time.
- Your LO followed a simple command.
- Your LO's vitals improved.
- Your LO read the menu and fed themselves.

- Your LO used the bathroom by themselves and used the call button to summon help.
- Your LO stood and balanced.
- Your LO took a few steps.

Caregivers, you can become the detective who looks for *evidence of progress*. As you do this you create a collective consciousness around your LO's healing. Progress may be slow, but if you want to maintain the hope and determination you'll need in this process of recovery, it's critical to keep looking for it.

Medical professionals are always concerned about giving people *false hope*. They believe they are tasked with giving information that helps people be realistic about their condition and their prognosis. In other words, *false hope* already presupposes there is *no hope at all* for recovery.

But let me address the topic of false hope through the story of just one couple, Thom and Karen.

I took Thom and his wife, Karen, to the doctor one week after Thom came home from the hospital. Thom was a 38-year-old father of 3 young children, who had suffered a catastrophic stroke that left him blind, agitated, impulsive, and speaking fluent nonsense due to Wernicke's aphasia. His wife was distraught and overwhelmed with caring for him at home.

At the doctor's office, she simply asked, "Is he going to get better?"

The doctor replied, "I don't want to give you false hope, he's had a severe stroke."

"If there's no hope, then why are we doing all these therapies?" she asked.

I was struck by the inaccuracy of the doctor's statement. *There is no such thing as false hope.* HOPE IS HOPE.

Hope is a feeling and a desire of expectation.

A doctor is justified in providing the facts of your condition, the results of the MRIs, the blood work, and so on, but hope does not show up on any lab report.

Hope is a belief, and all recovery, whether partial or full, begins with *belief*.

Did Thom get better? Yes. First, he recovered most of his vision, though he still had visual field cuts that caused him to neglect and often bump into things on his left side. Then his language and self-monitoring improved, and he could carry on short conversations. He became independent enough to walk to a neighborhood drugstore and complete a small transaction, including ordering and paying for an ice cream cone.

At the two-month mark of recovery, Thom's impulsivity had significantly lessened, and Karen thought he could safely stay home alone. Upon her return, however, when she didn't find him in the house, she followed the buzzing sound coming from the backyard. Thom was on a ladder trimming the palm trees with a chainsaw! Thankfully, he wasn't injured, but his impulsivity and poor judgement had her rethink some future home-*not-so*-alone strategies.

ESSENTIAL TAKEAWAYS

- Get out of the hospital gown and into rehab-ready clothes as soon as possible.

- Suit up, show up, start up, and stay consistent in your rehab routines.

- Fake it till you make it. Act as if you are what you want to be until you become it.

- Change your posture to change your mind. Sit or stand up tall.

- *HOPE is a belief that things can and will improve.* There is no such thing as false hope.

- Look for progress with a magnifying glass and magnify what you find.

HELP IS NOT A FOUR- LETTER WORD:
LEARNING HOW, WHO, & WHEN TO ASK (C)

13
CHAPTER

Even a lone wolf needs his pack.
~ Cara McLauchlan ~

We've obviously devoted a lot of time to talking about the care needed for a stroke survivor, however, now let's turn our attention to the caregivers reading this. Caregivers needs are often overlooked in the equation of support and care. Yet your well-being is of paramount importance because you are at the helm of this journey of recovery.

Caring for your LO may feel like a sacred privilege or an overwhelming burden, or a little of both, depending on your state of wellbeing and the moment. The emotional, mental, physical, and financial demands of caregiving can put strain on even the most positive and resilient person.

Many caregivers feel pushed to the brink of their limits, running the details of multiple lives and being responsible for every decision. Stress and overwhelm may be constant companions. Joy, relaxation, or even basic needs like a long, hot shower are ignored in deference to catering to everyone else's needs.

Despite desperately needing help, for many reasons caregivers may not feel comfortable asking for it. Caregivers may cycle through emotions of satisfaction, reward, frustration, anger, resentment, guilt, and remorse.

Asking for help may seem monumental, but in reality these four simple words can change everything: "Can you help, please?"

At some point in your LO's stroke recovery process, virtually every well-meaning friend or family member will say, "Let me know if there is something I can do." Many mean this, and giving a person *actionable* steps that require no thought from them can make them feel as if they have done something valuable and are an integral part of the "Recovery Team." In fact, they are.

> *Accepting help is actually a gift you give by allowing others the joy of serving.*

The most effective use of your limited time is assembling your Recovery Team.

You can simplify your life by designating key individuals to be the leads in varying roles, thereby giving you more time to manage the critical early stages of recovery with your loved one. In short, only you can be with your loved one and the doctors, but others can efficiently handle the daily activities needed to run other aspects of your life.

HOW TO ASSEMBLE A RECOVERY TEAM

There are three important questions to ask when choosing who will help you:

- Has the person offered?
- Are they capable?
- Do you and your LO want them to help?

Not everyone is right for the job even if they're the *obvious choice,* like your sibling, parent, or best friend—*even* if they've offered.

You intuitively know the person who will be efficient, effective, and add value versus the one who, despite their willingness, will add chaos, negativity, and neediness to an already stressful time.

Next, think about where these dependable people will help you the most. You are going to need a pit crew with a few specialties in the areas of:

- Food/Meals/Grocery Shopping
- Communication

- Home Care/Trash/Plants/Laundry
- Child Care
- Pet Care

READER CHALLENGE

Right now, while the thought is fresh in your mind and before you move on to the next activity, write down the names of three potential people who can help you.

GET SPECIFIC

Unless you want to end up with 20 lasagna casseroles and 15 Bundt cakes crowding your fridge, you're going to need to be specific. So how do you ask for what you need without seeming demanding?

Getting Specific with Groceries, Home, Child, and Pet Care

There are several free internet resources that help one create a system for organizing meals. They allow you to be specific about your food preferences, allergies, and special needs. In addition to creating a calendar of meal planning that all participants can see, some services even send email reminders before the volunteer's promised meal date to ensure coverage. Some of these services allow for other kinds of requests like rides, pet care, yard care, and/or child care. These websites are easy to navigate and, within a short period of time, can get your Recovery Team on a roll. Find out more information in Appendix resources under the category of Caregivers: Food.

If you are affiliated with a school or religious organization, you can ask for help there, too. Good, centralized coordination is key because support can sometimes be so plentiful that three people show up to bring your kids home from school or your doorstep ends up looking like a food bank.

Getting Specific with Communication: Keeping People in the Loop

Keeping family and friends informed can be a full-time job. Nonstop phone calls, emails, and text messages during which you repeat the same information can be draining and rob you of the time and energy you'll want to devote to being with your LO or taking a much-needed chill break for yourself.

Several options are available for having a centralized *private* space to share updates, ask for help, and get the word out about your LO's status and improvement. See the Appendix under resources for caregivers.

Why is centralized communication important?

- People generally want to support you physically and emotionally. Accepting their love and connection is very comforting and builds the momentum of belief in recovery. Designate a "social media" person who can dole out the information you want, in the manner in which you want. Consult with that person and edit the entries to make sure they're accurate and going to those you want. Sometimes this might include a daily or weekly update and may include pictures, if desired. Some social media sites specifically for caregivers can also set up a schedule of visitors with guidelines about visitation, like **no sick visitors**!

- Your LO can receive messages easily without having to communicate by phone or in person. Survivors always talk about how much they appreciate the love and support that comes by way of email, text or phone calls. Reading or hearing messages buoys their spirits and determination to recover.

- Weekly updates show progress and are helpful in allowing the survivor and the caregiver to see how far they've come when things look as if they've stalled or haven't progressed far or fast enough.

****A WORD OF CAUTION****

I recommend survivors *not* speak with work associates or employers in the early stages of recovery, especially not in writing and especially if aphasia is present. The medical condition of a stroke is so complex and fluid that erroneous conclusions about long-term decisions, like employment, can be made prematurely. A survivor's written mistakes that previously would have been ignored, like misspellings or grammatical errors, are suddenly looked at with a magnifying glass. People with brain injuries are scrutinized more than those without. Your LO has a right to their medical privacy. If need be, you as the caregiver can maintain contact with employers via phone so no written record exists.

Communication Tools:

- The usual suspects: Facebook, Instagram, Snapchat. Useful for information you don't mind broadcasting.
- Lotsa Helping Hands: *http://lotsahelpinghands.com*
- Caring Bridge: *www.caringbridge.org*.
- Group email or texts

Here is a link to a modifiable email template I've created for you to *Ask for Help*. Make it your own: *https://docs.google.com/document/d/1YWmYnzB7Qkl2GngdfQzifpaKTjgp2rELsSraT5vC7bQ/edit?ts=5a5d27ad*.

ESSENTIAL TAKEAWAYS

- Caregivers need help. They can't do it all. Accepting help is actually a gift you give by allowing others the joy of serving.
- Choose helpers carefully.
- Assemble a team to help with food, communication, and other household tasks.

- Use free online resources to organize helpers and communication. See the Appendix for websites that offer group sign-ups for food and communication.
- Use my modifiable email template (accessible by clicking on the link) to ask for help with specific tasks.

PART 2
What's Next?
Homecoming

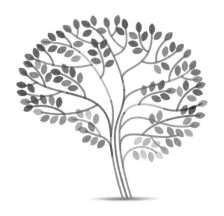

PREPARE FOR HOMECOMING *BEFORE* YOU LEAVE THE HOSPITAL (C)

The past is behind: learn from it.
The future is ahead: prepare for it.
The present is here: live it!
~ Thomas S. Monson ~

This is an exciting time for both the caregiver and survivor. You are about to make the transition from the hospital to home. Pause for a minute to appreciate all that that means. Now take a deep breath. While leaving the hospital marks the end of one phase, recovery is just beginning. There are a lot of moving parts to home recovery.

Returning home from the hospital is every survivor's dream. There is an underlying expectation that *all will be back to normal* simply because they've returned to something familiar. While home can, for some, be the perfect place to recover, it may not live up to the fantasy expectation. After all, it's not as if you've been on vacation and are returning home to jump into life as usual. Your LO is coming home with new needs that require adjustments from both of you. Things that were handled in the hospital, like using the bathroom, showering, dressing, eating, and even checking daily vitals like blood pressure, will require more time, equipment and involvement at home.

Everyone's routine will be "off." If your LO was the primary person responsible for running the household, they may likely be irritated with the condition of the house and its current state of functioning. Your LO's tolerance for noise and stimulation may be affected, especially if there are children and animals in the house. On the other hand, both children and animals can be a soothing balm of acceptance and love that aid in healing. Three things you will need for sure when your LO makes the transition home are flexibility, patience, and a sense of humor.

Before your LO is discharged from the hospital be certain that you, as the caregiver, feel prepared.

Hospital Tip: Hospitals are fined if a patient is readmitted within 30 days of discharge. Most rehab stays average 5.2 days. Insurance companies push for shorter stays and quicker discharges. Hospitals don't like fines or anything that dings their ratings. Be an aware consumer. If you're not trained and/ or prepared to have your LO come home because you feel they or you may be at risk for a rehospitalization due to medical instability or potential injury, tell your case manager you want your LO to remain hospitalized.

SAY THESE EXACT WORDS:

"I want (LO's name) to stay in the hospital, and I want you to please write my request and concern in the hospital records. I'm afraid if I take (LO's name) home, they will need to be rehospitalized because of (state the condition or concern). I want them to stay in the hospital until this problem is solved and we can go home safely."

Joon was a 6-foot-5, 38-year-old marketing executive with an 18-month-old daughter and a wife who stood 4 feet, 10 inches. Joon suffered a severe stroke at his office. I met Joon and his wife, Suki, at the hospital to see if he'd be a good candidate for our intensive home and community program. The hospital planned to release him in two days. Joon was impulsive, unsteady, and prone to anxiety attacks that made him leap to his feet and start stumbling around as he awkwardly tried to flee any room he was in. Apart from Suki's tiny frame and the caregiving demands required for her 18-month-old, their apartment had a 16-step entrance and 24 stairs to the bedroom. We convinced the case manager to hold off on discharge until modifications to the home entry were in place and a makeshift bedroom was made downstairs.

Larry was set for discharge in only three days, but he still had a *tracheostomy* (a hole in his neck creating a direct airway to breathe) and he required suctioning every couple of hours to prevent suffocation. His wife, Lisa, was willing to perform suctioning, but she was terrified, not only of the responsibility of that life-and-death procedure, but also because of Larry's many other nursing needs.

Lisa spoke the exact words I shared above when asking the case manager to extend Larry's stay. When they left the hospital many days later, Lisa was trained in suctioning, how to perform safe bed and wheelchair transfers, bathroom transfers, and how to monitor his oxygen tank and glucose. She practically earned a full nursing degree in a matter of days, and they both felt more secure upon homecoming.

Ideally your case manager will help prepare you for discharge. There are many things to think of before coming home. Inquire about the necessary items you'll need, like a hospital bed, commode (portable toilet), shower chair, etc. Work to have these items ordered and/or in place before your LO arrives.

If you think you will require a temporary or permanent disabled parking permit (or VIP placard!), download a DMV form at the link below and obtain the doctor's signature on the form. Please note, the link is for California's Department of Motor Vehicles, but each state should have a similar portal.

> *Do this before you leave the hospital—it's more complicated and time-consuming to do it later.*
> *https://www.dmv.ca.gov/portal/dmv/detail/forms/reg/reg195.*

If you have AAA, you can take the signed DMV form directly to their office and get a hang tag that day for a minimal fee.

Additionally, check with your LO's physical and occupational therapists to identify what equipment, if any, will be needed at home. Consult with the PT to learn how to adjust and use the walker, wheelchair, or cane, as well as how to disassemble and reassemble a wheelchair for transportation.

LOOK WITH NEW EYES

It's likely you've never had to look at your house through the lens of a person who's had some physical impairment, whether it was walking upstairs or even using the toilet or shower. You are either coming home with equipment and aids such as a wheelchair, toilet chair, shower chair, and a hospital bed, or you will need to order them.

How will you reconfigure your home to best accommodate your LO as they continue to improve and receive rehabilitative services?

First things first, how will your LO enter the house?

- Are there steps?
- Are there handrails?
- What kind of assistance will they need to enter the house?
- If they are wheelchair-dependent, can a ramp or lift be installed prior to homecoming?
- Will paramedics be required to transport the survivor inside the home and to various doctor appointments that will follow once they are living at home?

You must think about where and how they will sleep and use the toilet. Often a hospital bed is placed in the living room with access to a toilet nearby. Access to a bedside urinal is handy for men. Access to shower facilities are also important. Bath-only accommodations may require the purchase of a handheld shower nozzle and a shower chair for seated stability.

Ask Your OT and PT Questions to Prepare for Home Safety in the Bathroom

---

****A WORD OF CAUTION ABOUT BATHROOMS****

As previously stated, bathrooms are the single most likely location for a fall to occur. More people are hospitalized due to falls in a bathroom than from any other location. The hard and slippery surfaces in bathrooms may cause significant injuries to either your LO's limbs or head, resulting in further brain injury.

Falls are psychologically and physically not good for progress. Consult with your PT and OT for recommended safety items, strategies, and supervision levels your LO will need at home.

Equipment Safety

- Remove any slippery floor mats or rugs. Add rubber mats in the tub to prevent slips.
- Add grab bars in the shower. Consult with your OT or PT for proper placement.

Judgement Safety

If your LO needs bathroom help, *attempt to* agree on a rule about asking for help. Leave a bell or noise maker accessible for your LO to call if they need you. For impulsive types, put a small bell or jingling noise maker on their walker, so the noise alerts you or another caregiver if your LO is on the move.

Know the level of supervision needed. Learn the terms:

- Contact Guard Assistance (CG): A hand on the person to help stabilize them.
- Standby Assistance (SBA): Close by, but without touching.
- Supervised Assistance (S): Nearby, perhaps not even in the bathroom, but available to help if the person requests.

The most important thing to remember is this situation is *temporary.* Yes, this is disruptive. Hospital beds and rubber mats may not be the aesthetic you desire, but view it as temporary. The truth is things will either improve and your LO will be able to return to the bedroom and bathroom and their prior living arrangement, or a new plan will need to evolve. For now, take it day by day and remember that this is temporary!

WHAT NO ONE TELLS YOU, BUT YOU NEED TO KNOW

Coming home from the hospital is a great step toward recovery; however, the reality of being away from a medical facility equipped to handle emergencies may trigger a level of uncertainty or fear for both the LO and caregiver, especially if the stroke occurred at home. While your key focus after a stroke is on rehabilitation and recovering, understanding *why* your LO had a stroke is crucial for the simple reason that having one stroke puts them at greater risk for having another (recurrent) one.

The good news, however, is that 80% of strokes are preventable.

Here are the statistics, according to *Stroke.org*:

- Within 5 years of a stroke, 24% of women and 42% of men will experience a recurrent stroke.
- Recurrent strokes often have a higher rate of death and disability because parts of the brain already injured by the original stroke may not be as resilient.

These are tough statistics, but remember, **80% of strokes are preventable.**

REDUCE RISKS OF ANOTHER STROKE: MANAGE CONTROLLABLE RISK FACTORS

You can start reducing your risk of a recurrent stroke by managing the lifestyle factors you can control. These include:

- Managing blood pressure. Numbers should be 120/80 or lower.
- Keeping cholesterol levels in a healthy range of less than 200 mg/dL.
- Managing diabetes and sugar levels. Numbers vary throughout the day, so check with your LO's doctor to set their goal range.
- Be consistent and compliant with taking prescription medications.
- Quit smoking.
- Limit alcohol.
- Manage chronic stress through meditation and mindfulness.

- Eat a healthy diet with less processed food and red meat and more green and plant-based nutrition.
- Exercise regularly.

For an easy visual see the infographic on the last page of the book.

RECOGNIZE A STROKE AND REACT PROMPTLY

In the same way you should know what to do in case of any emergency, you should learn to recognize the symptoms of a stroke. Don't *anticipate* another stroke, but if you spot the symptoms in your LO, it's critical that you react promptly. Memorize the acronym in the infographic in the front inside book cover entitled "Recognize a Stroke."

Preserving brain function depends on time. Dr. Jeffrey L. Saver, a professor of neurology at the University of California, Los Angeles, calculated that for "every minute an artery is blocked, 1.9 million neurons die and the brain loses 14 billion synapses, the vital intersections between neurons."

The faster the diagnosis, the more options are available for preventing permanent brain damage. In an ischemic stroke (or blockage), the drug tPA can halt and even reverse neurological damage, but *only if administered within three hours from the onset of symptoms.* The more rapidly you respond to your LO's symptoms, the better their odds are for preserving neurological function and vital brain tissue.

ESSENTIAL TAKEAWAYS

- If you believe either you or your LO will be rehospitalized because of medical instability or injury, ask your case manager to extend their hospital stay until the problem is managed.
- Take inventory of your home and prepare it for your LO's ease, accessibility, comfort, and safety.

- Learn what mobility aids (orthotics, cane, walker, wheelchair) are being used or need to be ordered. Make sure the size and fit are correct.

- Learn to assemble and disassemble wheelchairs, walkers, or any other equipment needed for mobility. Do a practice run with your car.

- If your LO needs a disabled person parking placard, bring the DMV form to the hospital for a doctor's signature *before* they are discharged. Take it to AAA to obtain a placard the same day. California residents, click this link to download the DMV form for a handicap placard: *https://www.dmv.ca.gov/portal/dmv/detail/forms/reg/reg195.*

- Know the level of supervision your LO needs in the bathroom. Make sure grab bars, bath chairs, and non-slip surfaces are in place in the bathtub or shower.

- Get handrails, shower aids, and non-slip mats for bathroom safety.

- Know that your disruptive living arrangement is temporary. Make it functional and easy for everyone.

- Prevent a recurrent stroke by managing your controllable risk factors.

- Learn to recognize the symptoms of a stroke through the acronym FAST and react promptly. Rapid treatment for a stroke preserves vital brain cells and lessens potential damage. See the "Recognize a Stroke" infographic on the inner cover of this book . Memorize the FAST acronym.

A CAREGIVER'S GUIDE TO SANITY & REWARDING RITUALS (C)

15
CHAPTER

An empty lantern provides no light.
Self-care is the fuel that allows
your light to shine brightly.
~ Unknown ~

"Put your oxygen mask on first, then help your child." You've most likely heard flight attendants announce this during safety instructions. Why? It's presumed a conscious adult will care for their child more easily than a flight attendant caring for both an unconscious adult and a frightened child.

According to statistics from the National Alliance for Caregiving in collaboration with AARP, 23% of caregivers caring for a loved one for 5 years or more report that their own health is poor or fair. Many stop going to their own dental and doctor appointments. In addition, 40 to 70% of caregivers can suffer from depression. *It doesn't have to be that way.*

Simply put, you as the caregiver need to take care of yourself first, if you hope to care for your loved one with any degree of efficiency, competency, and sustainability.

With that in mind, you need to take time for a morning ritual.

I heard you laugh. I heard you swear at me, and I saw you throw down this book or rip the headphones out of your ears.

"You don't understand!" you scream.

You're right. I don't, but what I most certainly know is that *this short morning ritual is critical to your longevity, stability, and sanity.*

WHAT IS A RITUAL? HOW LONG DOES IT TAKE AND WHY DO YOU NEED IT?

A ritual could be a few things, and could last for as little as five minutes or up to one hour or longer. The point of the ritual is that it fortifies you, refuels you, nourishes you, and prepares you for the day.

This is coveted time and *must* be given to yourself.

It could be as basic as mindful breathing for five minutes or writing down three things for which you are grateful and really pausing to feel the gratitude. See Chapter 17: Managing Your Mindset and Finding Meaning for more information.

Rituals could be:

- Guided or unguided meditation set to a timer
- A walk or bike ride outside
- A run
- Stretching and yoga
- Any physical activity, especially dancing
- Reading, saying, or listening to prayer
- Listening to a spiritual message
- Journaling
- Visualization
- Mindfulness
- Focused breathing
- Tending to a garden

Whatever ritual you decide upon, you must commit to doing *something* daily that nourishes you. No one else can do this for you. The belief you must *do it all* may sometimes result in also inadvertently doing harm. A burnt-out, unappreciated, exhausted, and resentful caregiver is of no value to anyone. So make the promise right now, out loud, and say it three times, because no one else is responsible for caring for you but YOU.

*Affirm that: "Today I will take care of myself first,
because my wellbeing is my fuel."*

ESSENTIAL TAKEAWAYS

- Caregivers need daily rituals to maintain their wellbeing and be effective sources of help and support for their LOs.
- A ritual should be something that nourishes and restores the caregiver.
- It can be as brief as five minutes of mindful breathing or as long as an hour or more.
- If you don't make time to care for your health, your health will make time for you.

VISITORS & COMMUNITY REINTEGRATION (C&S)

16
CHAPTER

Visitors always give pleasure—if not the arrival, the departure.
~ Portuguese Proverb ~

Friends and family are critical to a person's recovery and sense of wellbeing, but too much of a great thing can be a detriment. It requires an enormous amount of energy for a survivor to be alert in the presence of a group, even if the survivor is not saying a single word. The noise and complexity of fast-moving conversation when multiple speakers are talking, sometimes simultaneously, in the presence of other background noise, such as music, cars, television, or kitchen noise, is extremely challenging for a person recovering from stroke. I can't stress this enough. Caregivers, even if your LO looks well and is enjoying the company, their brain is working extra hard, and you will see significant fatigue follow.

VISITORS: YOU'LL GET IT WRONG BEFORE YOU GET IT RIGHT

Initially, you will likely have too many visitors who stay too long. You will see how fatigued your LO becomes, and you can adjust accordingly. Generally, though, go with the mindset that less is more. You'll learn what works through trial and error, so pay attention to what length of time and how many visitors work best. Build in adequate rest time for your LO before and after having visitors especially if you are going on an outing later.

Set Visitors' Expectations Up Front

If therapists come to your home, make it known to visitors that therapy is your LO's job and first priority. Schedule visitors around therapy so they don't conflict. Here are some other ground rules your visitors should get acquainted with:

- Friends and family members who are ill should be asked to wait until they're well to visit.
- Limit the number of visitors at one time.
- Limit the time of visitation.
- Turn off all other noise sources when visitors are present.
- If your LO has eating or swallowing problems, opt for social visits without food.
- Allow for rest after a visit.
- Consider a visitor's presence as an opportunity for a break for yourself, unless you also want to visit.

Opt for Positive Visitors Only

People either bring light, energy, and support to a room, or they drain the energy out of it. It's detrimental to your LO to engage in stressful, combative arguments or to listen to sad and depressing news.

Protect your LO from negative people, if they can't do it themselves. There are always the *well-meaning* people who love sharing horror stories about people who've had strokes or other head injuries. *Keep negative people away,* or abruptly change the topic if they go on a rant.

You may sometimes have to choose between disappointing or offending a friend or family member and protecting and creating the optimum environment in which your LO can heal and recover. You and your LO will have to decide what outcome you want and who is more important in the long run.

If you still feel guilty, you can use the tried and tested doctor excuse. Blame it on the doctor, just like you blamed things on your parents when you were a kid. Politely tell the *Debbie Downers* wanting to come over that, "The doctor wants Jim to rest his brain for a while. I'll pass along your love and best wishes and let you know when he's ready for visitors."

Prepare Visitors for Emotional Changes

If your LO cries easily, explain that it's a common side effect of stroke. Tell your friends and family to ignore the outbursts and simply acknowledge your LO with the positivity that says, *I know you'll get through this.* Remain upbeat.

COMMUNITY OUTINGS

Community reintegration is a vital step in stroke recovery. It can be exhilarating, confusing, overwhelming, and a surprising adventure. How will you know if and when your LO is ready? For starters, ask them. The point of an outing is to get a person back into the community, and to do that, you just have to go for it. Sometimes a survivor may feel reluctant to go out in public. Feelings of shame, embarrassment, or concern that they may run into someone they don't want to see or talk to may prevent your LO from wanting to go out. If you can encourage your LO to go, it's best to start small. Think about a local environment that is not too stimulating or busy. A pleasant outing could be to a nearby park or library. Often the first outing is to the pharmacy to pick up medication. Plan your outing during an off-peak time and keep it to about 20 minutes or less.

Simple Tips for Outings:

- Appreciate the progress already made that enables you to be ready for an outing.
- Visit stores during their slow periods, like a supermarket at midmorning between Tuesday and Friday. *Avoid weekends and peak hours between 3 and 6 pm.*
- Use mobility carts that the store provides free of charge. Ask an employee to show you how to use one. Make sure your LO is capable of driving without crashing into things because of visual neglect or high impulsivity.

- Plan shorter outings (half an hour or less) at first, because even the car ride to get where you're going requires energy and will be fatiguing.
- If needed have a person of the same gender present to assist your LO in the bathroom. That said, many public places now have all-gender bathrooms, so if you and your LO are of the opposite sex, keep in mind that you may still be able to assist them.
- Check in with your LO to assess their level of comfort and fatigue.
- Make sure your LO has enough energy to return to the car.
- Have fun on your outing.
- Rest when you come home.

On your outings, you will discover some things you never could have predicted. You suddenly realize just getting from the parking lot into a store, even with a VIP (handicap) placard, takes more energy and time than anticipated. Public restrooms, even if accessible, are tricky to get into using one hand. You may find some environments are too stimulating with noise and bustling activity. Learn what works and what needs adjusting. Subsequent outings should encourage the LO's increasing independence, including talking with clerks, even if the LO has aphasia. Breaking the silence, acknowledging a challenge, and asking for help can aid survivors in making the leap to normalize their re-entry into the community. That's what happened with Maria.

Maria was a 36-year-old single mother of a teenage girl. Her stroke left her paralyzed on her right side and with severe communication problems. Although Maria understood everything anyone said, she had severe expressive aphasia. Maria was a stylish, beautiful young woman who'd mastered blow-drying her hair and applying the perfect thin sweep of eyeliner with her nondominant hand, but as persistent as she was in compensating for her motor skills, she avoided all speaking opportunities. She was ashamed and frustrated by her inability to "get the words out." She believed people, including her own daughter, thought she was "dumb." Early on I noticed Maria used her phone to text. When she was able to see this skill as a strength, she agreed to go to the supermarket with me.

Her task was to show a store clerk a wallet-sized card that said, "I've had a stroke and I have difficulty speaking, but I understand everything." After that, I suggested she use whatever communication means she wanted to get the clerk to help her in the produce department. Maria anxiously circled around the stacks of apples and oranges, often shaking her head "No" toward me. She even needed a second pep talk before she faced the challenge.

The clerk looked puzzled when Maria showed him the card, but as soon as he read it, he matter-of-factly told her she could always ask him for help. He even showed her the customer service area, telling her if he wasn't available others would gladly help her. Feeling more comfortable, Maria began typing on her phone, asking the clerk to pick out a watermelon and put it in her cart. By the time we left, Maria actually spoke a few words. She said, "Thank you," and told him her name. He acknowledged how "great" she was doing and said he looked forward to helping her again.

Once in the car, Maria burst into tears from the relief of facing her fear and finding out that people were not only not judging her as harshly as she judged herself, but they were also kind and affirming. It's true, some people may stare, but surprisingly the less you care, the less they stare. Focus on what you are doing, and you'll be great.

ESSENTIAL TAKEAWAYS

- Limit visiting time and the amount of visitors in your home, at least at first.
- Turn off noise distractions when visitors are present.
- Plan rest periods before and after visitors and outings.
- Opt for PPO: Positive People Only.

- Prepare visitors to ignore emotional outbursts and maintain positivity with support that says, *I know you'll get through this.*

- Community reintegration is a vital step in recovery.

- Plan a short local outing of about 20 minutes or less. A pleasant outing could be to a nearby park or library.

- Plan outings at off-peak times. Bring your VIP parking pass and plan to rest afterward.

- People may stare, but surprisingly the less you care, the less they stare. Focus on what you are doing.

- Use this link to download and print a *customizable* wallet-sized aphasia identification card: *https://theaphasiacenter. com/pocket-card/.*

MANAGING YOUR MINDSET & FINDING MEANING (C&S)

17
CHAPTER

Life is not the way it's supposed to be.
It's the way it is.
The way you cope with it is what makes the difference.
~ Virginia Satir ~

If only we could manage our thoughts as easily as we manage our visitors. Thoughts come to us at an astonishing pace—almost 50 thoughts a minute, adding up to a whopping 70,000 thoughts a day. Our thoughts create our feelings, which direct our actions, and ultimately create our results. While those thoughts may show up without our conscious consent, we do have a choice about *how* we respond to them. This chapter is for caregivers and thriving survivors who are ready to find meaning in the aftermath of a stroke.

PAYING ATTENTION TO HOW WE FEEL WILL TELL US WHAT WE ARE THINKING

If we know what we're thinking, we can make a choice to keep thinking it or reframe the thought in a way that may lead to a more positive outcome. You might say, "What else *could* I think about this stroke? It's horrible."

This is the point where I expect a lot of pushback, and I get it. Please know, I'm not telling you *what* to think. I'm gently, okay, maybe not so gently, encouraging you to examine your thoughts and listen to the narrative you're telling yourself.

Please trust me when I say that I'm not "blaming the victim" or being uncaring to your challenge. However, I am encouraging you to consider that it is *not* our circumstances, but what we *tell* ourselves about our circumstances that defines our feelings.

What are your story's main points and takeaways? Does your story have an ending? If so, what is it? When you feel ready, you may begin to compassionately and curiously ask yourself, "What else can this story be? What else can this story mean?"

I will repeat this:

> **It is not the circumstances, but what we tell ourselves about the circumstances that defines our feelings and influences our outcomes.**

How is this possible?

How could Tom Schumm, a newlywed of five months, say and mean, "My brain cancer is a gift," when he was told he had terminal brain cancer and was going to die in four to six months? His first response was not one of gratitude. He railed and raged against the injustice. Then, according to him, "amidst all the virulence came the inspirational voice of a very dear old friend, employer, and mentor, W. Clement Stone, one of the first to write about Positive Mental Attitude."

In his mind he heard him say, as he had thousands of times, "Every [a]dversity carries within it the seed of equivalent or greater benefit to those who have a Positive Mental Attitude!" Since Tom didn't have the option to live happily *ever after*, he weighed the choices of how he wanted to live his last few months of life. He reasoned that he could be bitter and angry and live in sorrow and isolation, or he could "[breathe] deeply and clearly," live contentedly and blissfully, and be remembered as a happy man of great courage. He reframed the *meaning* of dying by looking at how *he wanted to live*.

Tom's cancer was diagnosed in 2003, and in 2010 he published his story in *Chicken Soup for the Soul*, seven years after his terminal diagnosis. Even with the recurrence of his cancer in 2009, he chose to believe that cancer made him an "even better man the second time around." In 2018, Tom turned 70 years old. His current goal is "to live to 90, but if not, that's okay, too." In the meantime, he lives a daily life of gratitude, meaning, and contribution. On a side note, Tom says, "I had it easy, all I had to do was follow the doctor's orders." He credits his wife, Didi, with doing the research that allowed Tom to participate in an experimental trial back in the day when no viable treatments for brain cancer existed.

> Once again, whether it be cancer or stroke, it is not the circumstances, but what we tell ourselves about the circumstances that define our feelings and influence our outcome.

"How's that possible?" you scream. "This is a real event! My LO had a stroke and can't walk or talk, and can't work. Our lives are **devastated**."

You are right. The fact is your LO had a stroke. "Our lives are devastated" is not actually a fact. It is a *thought* you have about your life. You may be completely justified in *feeling* that, but it is not an objective fact.

Devastation may be your initial response, or even a longer-term response, but there are many survivors and their families who initially believed their lives were devastated, yet found meaning and purpose beyond what they ever thought was possible.

I expect that right now you might want to hurl this book at me and cry, "It's not your life!"

You are right. If I'm completely honest, I don't know how I would react. None of us knows what inner reserves or frailties we have until we are asked to activate them. I've certainly had my share of life's most difficult challenges, as we all do—mental and physical illnesses, addictions, eating disorders, financial losses, and traumatic deaths of people very close to me. Through these events, I've struggled, grieved, learned, and applied mindset tools to find meaning.

Most of us are quite familiar with the concept of posttraumatic stress syndrome (PTSS), but recently *posttraumatic growth syndrome* is gaining attention in research communities. Psychologists use this term to describe a *positive* change that occurs *after* an individual experiences a highly stressful life event. It suggests trauma does not have to debilitate a person. More importantly it recognizes an opportunity for growth where a positive transformation can occur.

Some survivors hear the word "psychologist" or "social worker" and dismiss their need for these services, by saying, "I'm not *crazy*." However, these highly skilled practitioners can be invaluable to help one manage mindset, find meaning, and gather badly needed but unknown resources. I encourage every survivor and caregiver to embrace the help of a social worker or psychologist.

I admit, I'm not an expert in the area of living with stroke, but my patients are. These people have *every* reason to call their lives devastated, and yet they find purpose, hope, resilience, and even joy in everyday situations. Does life still present challenges? Yes. Do they need to think more about accommodations than others? In some cases, yes, but not all. They view what's happened as a *new* condition and a situation that's manageable.

Typically at this stage of recovery my patients reach a pivotal point and we get deep. We get into the sadness, the anger, the frustration, and the fear. We look at what they are telling themselves this stroke means. When we keep asking, "What else could it mean?" or even "What's *good*? What can I appreciate about this stroke?" we often find light and a new perspective at the end of a very long list of ugly, horrible, wrong, and bad things.

Most people don't say, "I'm *glad* I had a stroke," though surprisingly there are quite a few who *do*, pointing out how the stroke woke them up to the radical changes they needed to make, including everything from relationships to work, to self-destructive addictions and behaviors.

For most, though, stroke is clearly not the life circumstance they would've chosen, but these survivors focus more on what they've gained than what they've lost. They report feeling loved at a depth never felt before. They share awareness of newfound kindnesses. Some appreciate how strong, determined, and "badass" they realize they are. Many develop new careers based on solving problems with products and services for which no one else had solutions. Their stories of triumph abound. You can read more of these stories in Chapter 25: Getting Your Life Back and Chapter 29: Conclusion: Forgiveness, Acceptance, & Reinvention.

Jean was one of those people whose life took an unexpected turn and then turned out unexpectedly. She was 49 years old and a Ph.D. level psychiatric nurse with a successful psychotherapy practice. She was a single parent of two daughters in their twenties. Jean's hemorrhagic stroke had a classic warning sign—a sudden, blinding headache—but sometimes even a healthy young nurse doesn't think *stroke*. The last words she spoke for a very long time were, "I feel funny."

Jean doesn't recall any of the details of the early hospitalization that took her from the ICU to an inpatient rehab program. Her kids refer to that period of time as her "never-never land phase." One thing Jean did remember, however, was thinking, "Oh, how easy and pleasant it would be to die." She said, "It just seemed to be fact."

Two sudden thoughts, though, abruptly catapulted her out of her "never-never land" and into the reality of *wanting to live*. The first was realizing that if she died, one daughter might be so upset she'd marry the boy Jean thought was no good for her and Jean wouldn't be around to influence her. The second thought was a feeling of remorse. The night before her stroke she and her other daughter had had an atypically angry phone argument, and they both hung up mad. Jean said, "I thought it'd be horrible if my daughter's last memory of me was an angry fight. There was *no way* I was going to die!"

That moment was a turning point for Jean. "From then on," she said, "I realized every time I opened my eyes, there was someone there whom I loved and who loved me. It was a level of love I had never felt before. I took it in so absolutely and so completely. That love was not just healing. It was lifesaving!"

Doctors didn't share Jean's *inner* enthusiasm for her life. A team case conference took place in her hospital room, with her doctor, family, and several nurse friends by her bedside. Although Jean's eyes were open and she appeared to be paying attention, she was mute. She hadn't spoken a single word since her stroke.

The physician opened the conference by saying, "Jean has severe brain damage and will, unfortunately, never again be able to care for herself or live independently, especially in her two-story condo. Jean is going to need long-term care. I suggest you sell her condominium to pay for her care."

Although Jean remained quiet, her family said, "Daggers were coming out of her eyes as the doctor spoke."

And then Jean said her first words: "NOT YET!"

What did Jean make her stroke mean? "It was the end of one life, but the beginning of another," she said. "It was also the beginning of my journey back to God. Despite having major physical disabilities including total right-sided paralysis, not speaking an intelligible word, not being able to read or do basic math, I understood everything. My cognitive skills were functioning. The parts of me I treasured most were the thinking and feeling selves, and they were still intact." See Chapter 29: Conclusion: Forgiveness, Acceptance, & Reinvention to read more of Jean's story and how she reinvented her life.

No conversation about finding meaning in life would be complete without speaking about Viktor Frankl, the psychiatrist. For three years between 1942 and 1945 he labored in four different Nazi concentration camps, including Auschwitz. During that time his parents, his brother, and his brother's pregnant wife perished. Based on his own experiences and the experiences of others, he later treated in his practice, Frankl pursued the question of how and why anyone survived the cruel unimaginable tortures, deprivations, abuses, and horrors of the Holocaust.

In his memoir, *Man's Search For Meaning*, he observed consistent patterns among survivors and discovered that *hope and meaning* were central to their survival. Frankl acknowledged suffering is unavoidable, but he stated there is "choice in how one copes with, responds to, and finds meaning."

Perhaps his greatest and most enduring insight is his observation: "*Forces beyond your control can take away everything you possess* except one thing, your freedom to choose how you will respond to the situation. You cannot control what happens to you in life, but you can always control what you will feel and do about what happens to you."

Frankl described three sources for meaning: Work—doing something significant; Love—caring for another person; and Courage in difficult times.

Managing your mindset is *not* **easy** work, but it is valuable.

WHAT'S THE BEST WAY TO MANAGE YOUR MINDSET?

The best way to manage your mindset is to be ahead of it. When it goes off the rails, learn to recognize it early enough. Pay attention to it. One mind-management tool is gratitude. Yes, gratitude at the most challenging time of your life. Don't take my word for it. Let's talk science.

Dr. Daniel Amen, a neuroscientist and psychiatrist who's performed over 10,000 MRI and spectrographic studies, observed the brain activity of people engaged in thoughts of gratitude and positive thoughts and compared them against those same people meditating on fearful anxious thoughts. Scans revealed seriously decreased activity in two parts of the brain when meditating on anxious thoughts compared with healthy brain activity when meditating on positive thoughts.

If gratitude is a little hard to swallow, think *appreciation*. Whatever we focus upon, we get more of.

Appreciation can start very simply. Look for small things to appreciate: a cup of delicious coffee, a prime parking spot, a smile from someone, a colleague who picked up a shift, a compliment received, a cheerful nurse, an answered call, a supportive friend, a chance to take a walk, a hot bath or shower, electricity, fresh water, or finding the exact resource at the right time. As we begin to stack up small appreciations, we warm our inner ovens and *feel* better. When we feel better, we take action from a more empowered and purposeful state of being. We become more resourceful and that leads us to better results.

> *Our thoughts create our feelings, which direct our actions that create our results.*

Sound familiar? I'll keep repeating it till it sinks in.

THE ROLE OF MINDFULNESS IN FINDING MEANING

The act of appreciation is a little like preheating an oven. You need a warmed oven if you want your cake to rise. Appreciation warms up your brain. Mindfulness and meditation are the full-on heat that bakes that cake.

Mindfulness simply means paying attention, but without thought. Sound confusing? Let me break it down. Mindfulness teaches us to notice our thoughts, but not analyze or dwell upon them. Each time you have a thought, you watch it pass without judgement, like an observer watching cars go by on a freeway. Thought after thought passes.

If you didn't already know, mindfulness helps you begin to notice how busy your mind is. But you breathe and allow it, without judgement. What's the point of this? Two things. First, when you are aware of your thoughts you can determine if they are *leading you* or *if you are guiding them*. Second, with practice and non-judgmental observation, eventually you will come to a place of spaciousness and quiet. It will likely be a fleeting moment at first, but long enough to notice the peace. Mindfulness is a novice's way to tiptoe into meditation.

Like anything else, the more you practice it, the better you will get. The single greatest health and life-giving tool you have is *managing your mind.* You do this by actively resting your thoughts and quieting your mind. It's free, and the only side effect is *peace and wellbeing.*

Dr. Deepak Chopra, a world-renowned pioneer in integrative medicine and the author of numerous books on healing, says,

"Meditation makes the entire nervous system go into a field of coherence." Chopra defines coherence as a highly ordered state of being, that is organized and efficient. "In a coherent system individual parts [operate] in harmony."

"I don't have time to meditate. I can't sit still, it's not for me."

You are not the first person to share these reasons why you can't and won't meditate. The question is, do you want to fight for your limitations or your limitlessness? Please know and understand that it's a choice. Both caregivers and survivors will benefit from mindfulness and meditation. I challenge you to do what is scientifically sound.

According to cardiologist Dr. Herbert Benson, "Any condition that's caused or worsened by stress can be alleviated through meditation." He is the founder of the Mind/Body Institute at Harvard Medical School's Beth Israel Deaconess Medical Center. Benson says, "The relaxation response [from meditation] helps decrease metabolism, lowers blood pressure, and improves heart rate, breathing, and brain waves."

There are apps and YouTube videos to guide you from one-minute mindfulness practices to an hour of meditation practice. Dr. Chopra and Oprah Winfrey have launched several free 21-Day meditation programs online. See Appendix Resources under Mental Health for Mindfulness and Meditation apps. Start with something simple and short. Practice daily and you will see benefits.

Rebecca was both a survivor and her own caregiver. She was the sole financial provider for herself and husband. Her husband had Alzheimer's disease and could no longer work. While Rebecca worked as a manager at a medical facility, her husband stayed at home with his male caregiver. When Rebecca's stroke landed her in the hospital for over a week, her husband's caregiver stayed in her house with her husband until Rebecca was discharged.

Rebecca lost her ability to speak and walk as a result of her stroke. During her hospitalization, she had no support from family or friends, and had to rely solely on herself to get better. Fortunately, her stroke symptoms resolved fairly rapidly. She recovered her ability to talk and walk well enough to return home. At home, though, is where an even greater problem unfolded. She began to suspect the husband's caregiver was stealing money as she watched her bank account dwindle. Even though her ability to do math was impaired, she could tell something wasn't right with her account. She was overwhelmed, scared, and still recovering, fighting fatigue and health issues.

When I began working with Rebecca, we first worked on making sure she was safe. The caregiver began to speak to her in ways that were psychologically and subtly manipulative, but because of her right brain stroke, the part of the brain that interprets non-verbal communication like tone, body posture, facial expressions and gestures, she couldn't exactly discern what was happening. Our agency provided her a social worker and an advocate for her protection.

The police ultimately verified that the caregiver was stealing money from her accounts and we helped her communicate with her bank to resolve the issue, but the day-to-day intensity of this experience wore her down and put her at great risk, until we did one small thing. We put an alarm on her phone to ring at three intervals throughout the day, at the times she identified she was most likely to feel stressed.

Rebecca chose a ringtone that was pleasant and different than any of her other alarms. We typed in a message to accompany the alarm that said, "I have the strength and stamina to keep going."

This daily mindset hack tamped down her anxiety and gave her the needed encouragement to keep going even when no one else was there for her.

A SIMPLE HACK TO HELP YOUR MINDSET

Send yourself a message. Most of us have smartphones these days. Set an alarm for the morning, afternoon, evening, and/or just before bed, or for the times of day you will most likely feel overwhelmed, frustrated, or anxious. Pick a novel ringtone and write a message that encourages. Write something like:

- You Can Do This
- Every Day I'm Making Progress
- I Am Doing My Best
- I Appreciate What I've Done
- I'll Find Meaning And Purpose In Everything I Do
- Everyday Gets Easier
- Everything I Do Profits Me
- I Will Keep Going No Matter What

The point is to write a message that inspires, supports, and nourishes you. Be your own loving coach. After a short period of time you'll be conditioned—yes, Pavlovian style—to hear that ringtone and feel a little better, breathe a little deeper, and stand a little taller. At first you'll find this boosts and surprises you, yet it's my prediction that it will support you at a deeper level than expected.

Jack was another survivor who needed a daily boost to laugh and relax. His personal alarm message said, "Find something funny and laugh!" This little encouragement re-sourced him back to the funny and light part of himself. This made him remember who he really was and what was really important. He said he could always find something to laugh about if he really tried— even something that might be considered humiliating, like missing the toilet in the bathroom when he was trying to stand. When he chose to laugh and see his progress through a *different* lens, he progressed more quickly.

What encouragement do you need?

What do you want your "coach" to say to help you believe you can keep going? You can find a new way. You can see things through a new lens. You can find something funny and laugh.

ESSENTIAL TAKEAWAYS

- Thoughts create our feelings, which direct our actions, that create our results.

- It is not the circumstances, but what we tell ourselves about the circumstances that define our feelings and influence our outcomes.

- Make managing your thoughts a priority.

- Manage your mindset with technology. Set regular, daily alarms with positive affirmations and messages.

- Make time for appreciation, mindfulness, and meditation. These free self-help healing tools have side effects: *peace and well-being.*

- Make appreciation or gratitude a daily practice. Write down three to five things for which you are grateful.

"TAPPING" DOWN ANXIETY, PAIN, & OVERWHELM (C&S)

"Everything you have ever wanted is sitting on the other side of fear."
~ George Addair ~

S troke survivors report feeling anxious a lot, even if they were never the nervous or "worrying" type before. In fact, about 20% suffer from some sort of anxiety disorder right after their stroke. Phobias and avoidance of situations account for the most frequent type of anxiety. Chronic anxiety in any form is bad for stroke recovery, as it keeps the body in an elevated stress response that inhibits healing.

Some anxiety after a stroke is normal. In reality, there are plenty of justifiable reasons survivors are anxious. People report increased worry about health, finances, work, and relationships. The uncertainty of what will happen can launch a person into thinking the worst. Learning about how anxiety works and what you can do about it should help lower that stress response and bring you to a more resourceful state of being.

WIRED FOR PROTECTION

The brain is wired, first and foremost, as a 24/7 security system to protect you. The *stress response* is what triggers the alarm that sets off a cascade of hormones. It begins in the *amygdala* (ah-MIG-dill-uh), a part of the brain that is one of the components of the *limbic system*. The limbic system is located in the midbrain, between the frontal lobes and the *hindbrain* (also called the reptilian brain—the most primitive part of the human brain.) The limbic system is the source of our emotions and long-term memory.

If this is a bit confusing, think of your amygdala, this tiny, almond-shaped network of neurons, like your computer's antivirus program. It's constantly scanning for anything that looks like, sounds like, or feels like a threat. If it finds a "match," it sends a signal to trigger the fight-or-flight response, also known as the stress response we talked about above.

The thing is, this "threat" setting off the amygdala's alarm bells doesn't have to be a real event. It can be an imagined one. The brain responds identically. That's why chronic negative thinking is so dangerous, because it keeps the stress response in overdrive, constantly raising glucose, adrenaline, and cortisol levels.

When the sympathetic system is on chronic alert, high levels of cortisol continue to course through your body, suppressing the immune system and creating oxidative damage to your arteries. *Chronic stress is devastating to the body and a potential trigger for subsequent strokes.*

Dr. Dawson Church, in his book *The Genie In Your Genes,* states, "Excess cortisol has been shown to reduce muscle mass, increase bone loss and osteoporosis, interfere with the generation of new skill cells, increase fat accumulation around the waist and hips, and reduce memory and learning abilities. Not only that, but over 1,400 chemical reactions and over thirty hormones and neurotransmitters shift in response to stressful stimuli."

Similar to posttraumatic stress disorder, some situations trigger more anxiety. For stroke survivors, whatever significant event happened *right before* the stroke, is often likely to re-trigger increased anxiety. For example, if the survivor had a stroke in their sleep, the *simple* act of going to bed could trigger anxiety that interferes with sleep.

Only a medical doctor can diagnose an anxiety disorder and separate it out from overactive nervousness that may be within your control. *It's important to seek medical attention if the anxiety is preventing you or your LO from functioning in life.*

Could your imagination be engineering your genes? "Yes," says Dr. Church. "A person performs his own epigenetic engineering on his cells in every instant with every feeling and every thought. When you understand that, you suddenly have a degree of leverage over your health and happiness."

For those of you who say you can't visualize, I challenge you to think again. Catastrophic thinking and fear are the greatest, most active forms of visualization, but regrettably the worst use of your imagination.

HOW YOU CAN "TAP" DOWN ANXIETY AND OVERWHELM

Emotional Freedom Technique, also known as "Tapping" is an evidence-based therapeutic tool recognized by the American Psychological Association that helps lessen anxiety, stop the stress response, and reduce the stress hormone, cortisol. It makes use of a technique that combines *Cognitive Behavioral Therapy* (essentially exposure and talk therapy) with *acupressure* (tapping on the energy meridians that run through our bodies).

What Does Tapping Do?

In short, it halts the stress response. Tapping turns off the amygdala's alarm, thereby deactivating the brain's arousal pathways. What's more, if tapping is done while experiencing or even discussing a stressful event, it reprograms the *hippocampus,* another organ in the limbic system that compares past threats with present signals and tells the amygdala whether the signal is a false alarm or a real threat.

Tapping allows one to bypass the conscious, thinking mind and get in touch with how the body interpreted and stored negative memories. The body stores memories primarily in four ways: visually, auditorily, kinesthetically, and through the olfactory sense of smell. Olfaction is our most ancient and primal memory store, and it's most closely linked to the limbic system.

Tapping is the tool that STOPS the FEAR response.

Tapping is also the tool that triggers the parasympathetic nervous system to turn on. This is commonly known as the *relaxation response.*

Your body essentially has two nervous systems that work like a teeter-totter. At one end, is the sympathetic nervous system; it is responsible for alerting you to fear and danger. This is a *very necessary* life-preserving system, as it allows you to take action and flee, fight, or freeze in a dangerous situation. At the other end of the teeter-totter is the parasympathetic system, known as the relaxation response.

The parasympathetic system is the *call off the dogs, all-clear, relaxation response* that triggers the release of DHEA, the most common hormone in the body, one that's associated with cell repair.

Tapping is a great self-help tool that can be used anywhere, anytime, and with great success and self-management. It has no side effects, except maybe self-consciousness because it "looks weird." That said, most everyone I've worked with would prefer temporary embarrassment to the side effects of addictive medications, if at all possible.

Use this link to learn how to tap: *https://youtu.be/pAclBdj20ZU.*

Tapping is not only useful for psychological issues, but can also be used for physical pain management.

Tapping is *not* a substitute for medical attention or intervention, but it is a useful tool in self-managing either chronic or episodic fear, anxiety, and pain, and it can be done anywhere and at any time.

Dario suffered severe pain from a *subluxed shoulder*, a common occurrence after stroke due to muscle weakness or spasticity in which the upper arm bone drops out of the shoulder socket. He was taking oxycodone to manage his pain. The medicine made him constipated and drowsy, but he needed it. In fact, just anticipating the pain he knew he'd feel when his meds wore off elevated his fear.

When Dario tapped, he successfully turned off his elevated fear and pain response. His pain ratings decreased from 10 down to 3. He was able to extend the time between medications and therefore required fewer pills overall. With less medication, he was more alert, and his constipation slowly resolved. Dario repeated tapping as often as he needed.

For some issues, tapping can be a "one and done" event, like it was for Maria. Maria was a postal clerk who enjoyed walking her route. She was normally very healthy, so she was alarmed by her unusually severe headache and dizziness. She entered an insurance company's office to drop off their mail, but felt so bad she asked to call the paramedics. By the time they arrived, Maria was having a seizure.

Although Maria didn't remember how she got to the hospital, she remembered awakening and seeing a doctor at the foot of her gurney. The doctor said, "Glad you're awake. We found a brain tumor. We don't know if it's malignant or benign, but we're running some tests and I'll let you know." He left her alone. Maria recalled the profound isolation and fear she felt.

When I met Maria at her home, she seemed to be recovering well. She showed me her list of medications. While we were chatting her sister walked over and held up a bottle of Ativan®. "Maria has panic attacks everyday near dinner time," she said. "It's very upsetting, she never had them before." Maria bowed her head, almost ashamedly, and acknowledged it was true.

I asked Maria if she wanted to stop feeling anxious and if she was willing to use a gentle technique that might help her reduce her anxiety and eliminate it completely. She was curious and agreed. I showed her the tapping points, and she followed along with me as I gently guided her. I encouraged her to change any words I offered into words that felt more accurate or resonant for her.

First, I asked her to think about the time of day she became anxious and to rate the intensity of it on a 0 to 10 scale. Ten was the most anxious and zero meant there was no concern or intensity at all. As Maria got in touch with how she felt (what visual images she saw, what sounds she heard, and how her body felt), she rated her intensity at a 10.

We began tapping, using a four-fingertip percussive tapping approximately four to seven times on the body parts shown on the following image with the set-up statement: "Even though I don't know why I feel anxious, I accept myself and am willing and open to finding peace." We said that statement three times as we tapped on the "karate chop point," also known as the point of psychological reversal.

We then tapped on all the body points listed on the chart below, while using a variation of the set-up phrase. As other thoughts came, we followed the intuitive unwinding and tapped on those thoughts, too.

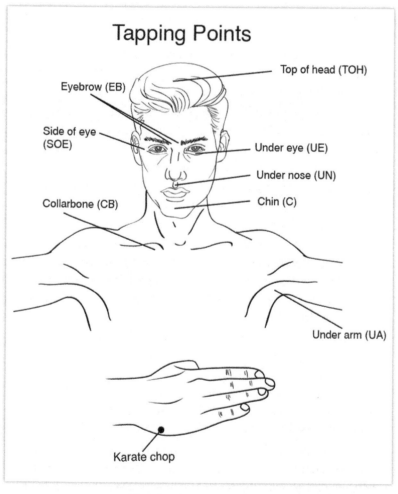

Tapping Points

- Eyebrow (EB)
- Top of head (TOH)
- Side of eye (SOE)
- Under eye (UE)
- Under nose (UN)
- Collarbone (CB)
- Chin (C)
- Under arm (UA)
- Karate chop

Meridian Tappping Points

Tapping Sequence and Statement Script

Eyebrow: This anxiety

Side Eye: This fear

Under Eye: This terrified feeling

Under Nose: I'm so alone

Chin: So scared

Collar Bone: This fear...

At this point Maria said, "I just noticed something."

"What?" I asked.

"I remember when the doctor left, I felt so alone and all I could hear was a loud ticking of the wall clock."

"What time was it?" I asked.

She burst into tears. "Five o'clock," she said, suddenly recognizing where and when this anxiety developed.

We tapped some more, but at this point Maria's intensity level had dropped to a zero and she felt an enormous sense of relief. Maria never had another panic attack during her course of recovery. She still had to manage a challenging course of physical and cognitive recovery, but she was able to do it without the paralyzing fear that always set her back.

Rob was an 83-year-old man with a keen sense of playfulness. If he wasn't hiding plastic ants in his wife's salad, he was shooting soft rubber bands at her feet to get her to dance. Rob was a well-read and well-travelled man who loved football, investments, and race cars. His stroke left him with moderate aphasia that made communicating difficult. His reading skills were also severely affected. Although he read and understood the symbols needed for executing trades for his online investments, he found it impossible to read books or his prized race car magazines.

Rob had a problem. He had to renew his driver's license. At his age he had to pass both a driving and written test. The driving portion didn't concern him. He knew he was a good driver, and he had proof from the occupational therapist who assessed him. He'd passed his "practical driving" exam with flying colors, but his written test loomed ahead.

Reading is often impaired after a stroke. By the time Rob got to the end of a sentence, he'd forget what he'd read. Reading was a word-by-word experience, it was no longer automatic or holistic. It was like having lots of little pieces of a puzzle but not being able to put them together.

We spent many sessions reading questions aloud from the DMV manual. He followed along by pointing to each word and then listened to the whole sentence. Finally, he practiced taking tests online to train both his eyes and his ears to understand the sentence as a whole.

While Rob demonstrated competency for his online test, we knew testing at the DMV would be another challenge. There would be many distractions and lots of noise, plus the pressure of wanting to pass caused him increased anxiety. Anxiety and fear never help the brain find resourceful solutions. *Fear* is the trigger for the brain to flee, fight, or freeze—none of which are useful when trying to pass a written test.

To accommodate this fact, Rob made an appointment at the DMV for an off-peak time. He advised his examiner that he'd had a stroke and it was difficult for him to talk, but he understood everything. He showed the examiner the results of his OT evaluation who tested not only his driving skills on and off the freeway, but also tested his knowledge of road signs and speed limits and his cognitive skills of memory, judgement, and problem-solving. (See Chapter 26: Driving & Working for more information on driving evaluations.)

In the mornings and evenings preceding his test, Rob and his wife, Judy, used the tapping scripts I wrote for them. Judy read the words while he tapped and brought down his stress response. At the DMV, Rob took his time and used a reading ruler to keep his vision tracking on the line he was reading as it had a tendency to jump to other lines.

When the DMV clerk stamped his approval for a renewed license, Rob was elated, proud, and relieved. This major accomplishment was a key to his freedom. He felt a sense of independence and contribution. Now, Rob enjoyed solo trips to the pharmacy knowing he could talk with the pharmacist at his own pace. It gave him a chance to wander the card aisle and find the right sentiment for his wife. Driving allowed him to feel as if he was contributing by going to the market for his wife or by taking turns at the wheel on their long trips to the desert. Driving boosted Rob's self-esteem and gave him the feeling of wholeness he'd been missing.

HOW TO TAP

- Learn how to tap and learn the tapping points with this Tapping for Beginners video: *https://youtu.be/pAclBdj20ZU.*
- Obtain a free mini-manual about Emotional Freedom Techniques (EFT, or tapping) and how it can help: *www.eftuniverse.com*
- Get the Tapping Solution App (free on Apple, not yet available for Android). Visual and verbal instructions and rating scales are provided. Progress is tracked. *Some tapping sessions for anxiety are free.* Although free to download, monthly and annual fees apply to access the full menu of monthly changing scripts.

ESSENTIAL TAKEAWAYS

- The American Psychological Association (APA) recognizes tapping as an evidence-based, accepted practice of therapy for reducing anxiety and pain.
- Tapping combines Cognitive Behavioral Therapy with Acupressure meridian points on the face and chest.
- Anyone can perform Tapping, even if one is paralyzed on one side of the body.
- Tapping lowers stress levels and improves wellbeing.
- Tapping can lower pain and anxiety and may lead to a reduction or elimination of medications used to treat

these conditions; however, *it is not a substitution for medical evaluation or treatment.*

- EFT practitioners, Tapping scripts, and videos are available online. (See the Appendix for resources under Mental Health.)

- Always seek medical attention from a physician if anxiety is excessive, persistent, and interferes with normal life activities.

- Learn how to tap and learn the tapping points with this Tapping for Beginners video: *https://youtu.be/ pAclBdj20ZU.*

- See the Appendix under Mental Health for information about the Tapping Solution App.

GETTING ON AUTOPILOT (C&S)

Motivation is what gets you started.
Habit is what keeps you going.
~ Jim Rohn ~

THE "SECRET" SUCCESS OF ROUTINES

Routines are important for conserving energy and brain power. The fewer decisions one makes the more brain energy one has to accomplish the more challenging cognitive and motor tasks that are part of recovery. To begin, let's talk about how a routine, procedural memory and habits are different.

Routines are any activities we do in a regular and predictable sequence. Think of a morning routine that follows a consistent pattern of activities: wake up, shower, read the paper, eat breakfast, and work out.

Procedural memory is that part of our memory that allows us to automatically perform activities without thought, for example, tie our shoes, brush our teeth, make a cup of coffee, get dressed, and manage our phones, because we've mastered the individual steps required to perform these activities. We don't have to consciously think each element.

After a stroke, procedural memory is often intact for many "routine" activities, but sometimes what was routine *before* is no longer routine. It's the conscious act of learning or relearning that takes the activity out of the realm of the automatic. It is anything but routine to learn how to make paralyzed limbs wake up and "relearn" how to move, balance, walk, or grasp, or to teach a nondominant hand to *learn* to blow-dry hair, put on makeup, zip a zipper, or write.

These tasks require more brain power and more focused energy, which always translates to more fatigue.

We create habits through the small decisions and actions we take every day. In other words anything we do repeatedly creates our habits. James Clear, the author of *Atomic Habits*, says, "All habits have a 3-step pattern: Reminder (the trigger that initiates the behavior), Routine (the behavior itself; the action you take), and Reward (the benefit you gain from doing the behavior)." Sound familiar? Repetition of behavior is *neuroplasticity at work*, and it can be used to your detriment or advantage as you will see later in this chapter.

The value of creating a predictable routine, i.e. *schedule*, is to conserve the caregiver's and the survivor's brain power, improve memory, and increase the survivor's self-regulation and independence.

I've watched families thrive with the simplicity of a schedule because they knew what to expect. They utilized their energy for activities that encouraged progress and wellbeing, rather than draining themselves through energy-sucking activities like calling and emailing people to change appointments and redo schedules.

My observation is that the families who adhere to routines, as best they can, do far better and have less stress than those who don't. Higher stress and slower progress are more likely outcomes when schedules are haphazard and unpredictable and when there is an open-door policy for drop-in visitors.

The stroke survivor gains greater self-esteem, competency, self-regulation, and a feeling of normalcy when they feel more in control and aware of what to expect.

Whether you're a caregiver or a survivor, first and foremost, you're a human being. Morning rituals are the foundational practices of some of the most successful human beings on the planet. But *what* goes into your morning ritual is what sets the tone for your day. What you choose matters.

REWARDING RITUALS: KEEP IT SIMPLE

The Miracle Morning by Hal Elrod shows how a morning routine built around six key practices known as "Life S.A.V.E.R.S."— silence, affirmations, visualization, exercise, reading, and scribing (journaling)—helps you get more done and live your best life.

Your morning is the most likely time you'll have control of the events of the day to the extent that you can include a ritual of gratitude, mindfulness, and some form of exercise. These three things take 15 to 30 minutes, but doing them regularly will have an enormous impact on establishing the tone for your day. Hey, if you're up to Hal's suggested six things, go for the gold! This may mean waking up 30 minutes before other household members arise, especially if there are children present and a hectic school schedule needs to be met.

Establishing the plan and setting up the environment the night before leads to what I call *inevitable* success.

HOW TO MAKE YOUR PLAN OF ACTION *INEVITABLE*

Get to know your LO's level of cognitive function and language skill to determine the degree to which they can participate in planning your morning routine. Initially, they may only be able to follow immediate commands about forthcoming events in the routine. Nonetheless, your LO should be offered the dignity and respect of being shown and told the daily schedule, including external reminders (phone alarms or a daily schedule) for frequent reference. Short-term memory challenges may mean you will need to repeatedly remind them of what's happening next.

Ideally, the LO can be trained to use their own external reminders, like a smartphone or other personal assistant, and develop the habit of asking, "Hey Siri, Alexa, or OK Google, what's my schedule for today?" ** Hint: You may have to post the name of the device in several locations as it's common for stroke survivors to have difficulty remembering and retrieving names. Without that name, they won't be able to activate the device.

Here are some more tips to make your success inevitable:

- Do the same things in the same order every morning, so the routine becomes *routine;* this is a key to conserving brain energy and not succumbing to decision fatigue.

- If your LO can select their own clothes, make sure they're laid out the night before so getting dressed is quicker. Not only does it make the morning go more smoothly, but it primes the brain, before sleep, with the right message: **I'm in recovery mode. I'll get dressed and be ready.**

- If you or your LO are writing in their stroke recovery journal make sure it's *always* in the same place with a selection of sharpened pencils. It's better to write than to spend your writing time searching for supplies.

- The morning ritual of writing in the journal while sipping coffee or tea is a great way to jumpstart your mindset. It's the first "therapy" of the day, tackling the skills of memory, writing, visualizing, and affirming.

- Practice mindfulness. Have your timer handy and whatever phone app, video, or audio recording you prefer to establish a 5 to 10-minute mindfulness practice. This is a time for quiet reflection to observe your thoughts without judgement. Some prefer this time for a daily Bible ritual or to read or listen to uplifting messages. Whatever activity connects you and your LO to a dedicated period of quiet reflection is scientifically proven to enhance focus and elevate the body's own repair mechanisms by creating the right hormonal brain activity. See the Appendix under Mental Health for Mindfulness and Meditation Apps.

- Practice appreciation or gratitude. Write down three to five things you can genuinely appreciate that cause you to feel good when you think of them.

- Exercise. Do you have a written plan from the PT or OT? Are you following along with a YouTube video or other program? Whatever it is, make sure your body is in motion.

Dr. James Levine of the Mayo Clinic says, "The chair is out to kill us. Sitting is the new smoking." Get a Fitbit that vibrates when you've been sitting too long as a reminder to get up and move. Doctors, physical therapists, and fitness trainers all say that if exercise were a pill, it would be the most prescribed and beneficial drug in the world.

MENU OF ACTIVITIES

It's a huge sign of progress psychologically and cognitively when your LO is ready to start planning their day. Psychologically, because it means your LO has a purpose and reason for getting up and because they are exercising a degree of control and management about their life. Cognitively, because planning and scheduling are complex executive skills requiring memory, language, a conceptual awareness of time, and the ability to visualize and anticipate future events.

How can a menu of activities help? Just like a restaurant menu helps you decide what you might like to eat, a menu of activities helps your LO whose language or memory may be impaired conceptualize and choose an activity in order to help plan their day.

New ideas may be added as your LO's skills and abilities improve. If reading is impaired, create a menu with pictures.

Generating a menu with three categories, mental, physical, and leisure/spiritual, is a good start. (See the Appendix under Caregiver Resources for a link to a blank template for a "Menu of Activities." Below is an abbreviated example.)

MENTAL	PHYSICAL	SPIRITUAL/ LEISURE
Word puzzles	Perform P.T. Exercise program	Meditate
Cognitive games/ Apps	Walk in neighborhood	Listen to music
Write in journal	Chair yoga	Read bible/ Listen to spiritual positive messages

20

Every day should involve *some* focused activity. It doesn't have to be *equally* balanced among mental, physical, and leisure, but a weekly schedule should have elements of each area to fulfill these three basic human needs.

Whatever we do repeatedly and consistently will change our brains.

I want to repeat this because, as you know, repetition is the basis of *neuroplasticity*.

Whatever we do repeatedly will change our brains. Our brains will build more efficient pathways on the basis of repetition. This is true for both positive, desired outcomes as well as those less desired. These repeated behaviors become our habits. If we continue to lie in bed and passively watch TV, our brains will accommodate to passivity. We will become less efficient at activity or verbal engagement. Our habits determine our daily outcome, which in the end determines our lives.

Learned dependency and depression are very real saboteurs of recovery

Learned dependency or helplessness may occur because of two factors. First, it may occur because the LO feels they have no control over their situation. Second, because a caregiver may *overhelp a* LO for a variety of reasons including: a sense of love, fear, duty, guilt, their LO's demands, or because it's simply easier and faster. However, when we do *everything* for a survivor and don't allow opportunities for struggle and growth, we rob them of developing skills and unknowingly give them the message that they are not and will never be capable. It's true, it's harder and slower for everyone to allow the LO to take their time and figure out and perform whatever it is they are trying to achieve, but the long-term gains of self-sufficiency and self-esteem are worth it for everyone.

Do Nothing, Go Nowhere

We all love an occasional "do nothing, have no plans" kind of day, but the risk of becoming depressed is tremendous if a person has no plans, nothing to anticipate, and nothing to accomplish. Stroke recovery is definitely about USE it or LOSE it. It's virtually guaranteed that this state of passivity and dependence will lead not only to depression, but a worsening of every marker of recovery. Walking and motor functions will dissipate. Memory and engagement will diminish. Depression is real, and without the draw of an activity or stimulation other than passively watching TV, recovery can dramatically slow down and gains can be lost.

DEPRESSION

Clinical depression is a common side effect of stroke. It affects one in three people at some point within the first five years after a stroke. According to the National Institutes of Health, post-stroke depression is underdiagnosed. Consulting a doctor for a diagnosis is important to differentiating between episodic sadness and true clinical depression.

While it is normal (though of course not desired) to feel sad and worried after a stroke, as mentioned earlier, stroke has a way of "turning up the volume" on behaviors and personality traits that existed before the stroke. Whatever personality traits a survivor exhibited prior to the stroke are likely to be more intense after the stroke. If your LO suffered with clinical depression prior to stroke, it's likely to be exacerbated.

If either you or your LO is suffering from a persistent sadness, withdrawal from family and friends, an inability to initiate, and a degree of emotional flatness that interferes with life, you need to seek the assistance of your doctor.

This is not to be confused with the teary-eyed emotional vulnerabilities your LO may express. It's common for survivors post-stroke to be more emotional, more vulnerable and weepy. Even the most stoic, tough-as-nails men are prone to displays of deep emotion. While this may be uncomfortable for them and their loved ones who are not used to seeing such emotion, it is a feature of post-stroke recovery.

This behavior is different from pseudobulbar affect (PBA) where emotions are volatile and changeable and have no apparent or appropriate connection to the situation. In this condition a person may laugh or cry at inappropriate moments and for no obvious reason. Your doctor can make the differential diagnosis and prescribe the right medication for PBA.

A thorough medical evaluation is needed to diagnose and treat depression. While there are numerous medications for depression, it's important to evaluate simple things that might contribute to depression, from sleep schedules to food, to physical activity. Implement simple, common-sense measures before choosing to medicate your LO to see if these changes have positive effects. These could include adding meaningful, purposeful activities that appeal to your LO, like animal care, adaptive gardening, or other types of volunteer work.

Because there are many classes of antidepressants, each with their own unique features, finding the right "cocktail" is as much an art as it is a science. If you or your LO use medications to manage depression, work closely with your doctor and report symptoms of improving or worsening feelings. Every medication carries some side effects, and while some are quite minor and worth the improved state of wellbeing, others are not. Be willing to experiment to find the right medication and give it time to work. Antidepressants typically take up to two weeks or more before noticeable differences are felt and seen. The risks and benefits for using medication must always be weighed; however, the risks of not treating depression can also lead to dire outcomes.

Dr. Dolores Malaspina, director of the psychosis program at Icahn School of Medicine at Mount Sinai Hospital, New York, says, "Untreated chronic depression and long-term stress inhibits synaptic formation, thus inhibiting recovery and resiliency." She cites encouraging medical research that suggests antidepressant medications may induce both *neurogenesis* (the formation of new neurons) and *synaptogenesis* (new synapses) that contribute to the brain's structural and functional plasticity. She strongly recommends, "People suffering with depression should seek treatment for the best outcome."

Experimentation, time, careful monitoring, and observation are necessary to determine if a drug is working. How will you know? Are you or your LO more engaged? More willing to participate in activities? Demonstrating more variety in emotions? Improving or regulating your eating?

You must always consult your doctor if you want to stop taking medication. Consult your doctor for strategies in *easing off the drugs* to prevent serious side effects. *No* antidepressants should be stopped suddenly unless indicated by your doctor. Medication alone may or may not improve mental outlook. For a more comprehensive approach seek counseling with a psychologist or social worker to include behavioral strategies to improve mental wellbeing. For a self-help non-medicinal approach to reducing stress and anxiety and improving mental wellness, see Chapter 18: "Tapping" Down Anxiety, Pain, & Overwhelm.

ESSENTIAL TAKEAWAYS

- Routines are important for conserving energy and brain power.
- Daily rituals of writing, quiet reflection, gratitude/appreciation, and exercise scientifically improve brain function and aid in positive recovery.
- Plan daily routines to include three types of activity: Physical, Mental, & Spiritual/Leisure.
- Make success for completing activities *inevitable* by creating the environment to support it. For instance, set up clothes and items needed for activities the night before.
- Depression affects one in three people at some point within the first five years after a stroke. According to the National Institute of Health, post-stroke depression is underdiagnosed. Talk with your doctor if depressive symptoms are persistent and interfering with recovery.

- Depression and learned dependency will sabotage recovery.
- Always consult your doctor before stopping medications, especially antidepressants. You must slowly be weaned off of them to prevent serious side effects.
- Seek counseling with a psychologist or social worker as a part of the behavioral approach to mental wellbeing.
- For a self-help non-medicinal approach to reducing stress and anxiety and improving mental wellness, see Chapter 18: "Tapping" Down Anxiety, Pain, & Overwhelm.

THE *SIMPLE* MATH FORMULA TO NUTRITIONAL WELLNESS THROUGH FOOD (C&S)

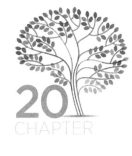

20
CHAPTER

Your fork is the most powerful tool to transform your health.
~ Mark Hyman, M.D. ~

If we are what we think and we are what we speak, then we certainly are what we eat.

It's not that complicated—wellness requires simple addition and subtraction. *Add* food and substances that improve your health. *Subtract* the stuff that stops or inhibits wellbeing.

Let's look at the fundamental math formula for nutritional wellness:

Add: Water and healthy food.

Subtract: Substances that clog your arteries, cause *inflammation,* and jack up your blood sugar (glucose) and blood pressure.

Harvard Health Publishing explains that when your immune system is healthy it defends against invaders that threaten it, such as "invading microbes, plant pollen, or chemicals." This triggers a process called inflammation. Not all inflammation is bad. It is a sign of good health to have intermittent bouts of inflammation as long as it's directed toward true invaders. The problem is when inflammation becomes a chronic, day in and day out occurrence. Inflammation is the culprit linked to many major diseases including cancer, heart disease, stroke, diabetes, arthritis, depression, and Alzheimer's disease.

What causes inflammation? Bacterial infections, viruses, emotional stress, physical stress, insulin resistance, allergens, and common foods that are typical of the Standard American Diet (SAD).

The most common foods that inflame include:

- **Sugar and high fructose corn syrup.** Read your nutritional labels. Virtually every substance listed in the ingredients of packaged food ending in "-ose" is a form of sugar (sucrose, glucose, fructose, lactose, etc.). Sugar is present in **cookies, candy, ice cream, and sodas.** Sugar may also counteract the good, anti-inflammatory effect of omega-3 fatty acids.

- **Artificial trans fats.** Ingredients labeled as "partially hydrogenated oil" are *bad for you.* They're in **margarine, shortening, lards, and most processed foods.** Ironically while they're used to extend the shelf life of the product, they act to threaten your life.

- **Vegetable and seed oils (including sunflower, safflower, canola, sesame, and peanut).** These highly processed oils are often extracted from foods using solvents like hexane, a component of gasoline. They have a high omega-6 fatty acid content associated with inflammation. (We need more omega-3 fatty acids and fewer omega-6.) **Fast foods and fried foods** are typically made with these oils. Read your labels.

- **Refined Carbohydrates.** These include **white breads, white rice, pasta that is not whole grain, bagels, pastries, donuts, cereals, pretzels, chips,** and any product where the fiber is removed and the food is highly processed. Refined carbohydrates raise blood sugar levels and may encourage the growth of inflammatory gut bacteria that can increase the risk of obesity and inflammatory bowel disease.

- **Red meat and processed meat.** Common types of processed meat include s**ausage, bacon, ham, smoked meat, and beef jerky.** Processed meat is high in inflammatory compounds like advanced glycation end products (AGEs). AGEs are formed by cooking meats and some other foods at high temperatures.

- **Excessive Alcohol Consumption.**

YOU *CAN* PUT OUT THE FIRE OF INFLAMMATION

Lindsey Layton, a certified wellness coach from the Institute of Integrative Nutrition, says, "We basically want to 'put out the fire' of inflammation by eating foods that reduce it, including clean, unprocessed foods that are consumed closest to the garden." She says, "If I can't pick it off a tree or pull it out of the ground, I probably shouldn't eat it!"

Foods that put out the fire of inflammation (anti-inflammatory foods) include:

- **Extra virgin olive oil, coconut oil, flaxseed oil, fish oil**
- **Green, leafy vegetables**, such as broccoli, cauliflower, spinach, kale, and collards. ***You may need to avoid or adjust your consumption of these if on blood thinners***
- **Avocados**
- **Mushrooms**
- **Tomatoes**
- **Nuts** like almonds and walnuts
- **Fatty fish** like salmon, mackerel, herring, anchovies, and sardines
- **Fruits,** especially berries, like strawberries, blueberries
- **Green Tea**
- **Turmeric,** a spice used in curries combined with black pepper (can be found in supplement form).
- **Dark Chocolate containing at least 70% cacao.** *(Not milk chocolate that's loaded with sugar.)*

We all want a simple answer, yet when given one it's often dismissed as too easy. Let's not confuse easy and simple. Simple is the least complex, the most basic, and perhaps the most common-sense, but certainly not common practice. Simple does not mean it's "easy" to do. Just drinking six to eight glasses of water a day when you previously drank sodas, coffee, and juice is not necessarily an *easy* behavioral change, but it is *simple*.

Simple Addition #1

Drink more water daily.

Our bodies are approximately 60% water, and our cells need water to perform every function. Water is to our cells what batteries are to a flashlight. No battery power, no function. It takes only 2% dehydration to negatively affect your memory, attention, and other cognitive skills.

So how much water does a person need? The average is based on weight and height, but without making it too complicated, aim for drinking between six and eight 8-ounce glasses of water per day.

How do you tell if you are not getting enough?

Your urine will be dark yellow. Taking vitamins may turn your urine a brighter shade of yellow/green, but dehydration turns it darker yellow, verging on amber brown.

This basic addition to your life can make a substantial difference in energy, in synaptic firing, in blood pressure regulation, and even in your medication's effectiveness.

How do you make this simple addition to your life *inevitable?*

Have a pitcher of water set up the night before. Make it interesting and fun by adding some taste enhancers. Get creative and add one or more of the following: lemon, mint, orange slices, cucumber, green tea bags, or any other fruit or herb that might make it more interesting to drink.

Buy 16-oz. recyclable bottles and always have them handy. Aim to drink four a day.

Juice, soda, and coffee are not the same as water. Juice adds a lot of sugar to your diet and changes the chemistry of your glucose. Sodas and especially diet sodas are concoctions of sugar, sodium, and chemicals that are dangerous. Sodas are on the *subtraction* list. That is not to say never drink one; however, if your habit is to drink three or more sodas a day, the sheer amount of sodium is likely wreaking havoc on your blood pressure. Learn to read food labels and do your best to subtract from your diet anything with artificial colors, flavors or preservatives.

Simple Addition #2

Choose fresh fruits and vegetables and you won't have to read labels! Add *nutrient-dense* food. Think of nutrient dense food like *more bang for your buck* food. That is, it is loaded with vitamins, minerals, nutrients, and enzymes necessary for the body's cellular regeneration. The more nutrient-dense foods you consume, the more satisfied you will be with fewer calories. Nutrient-dense foods are typically those found in a wide variety of vegetables and fruits.

If you want to know how your food stacks up, consult the ANDI score (Aggregate Nutrient Density Index): *www.drfuhrman.com/ content-image.ashx?id=73gjzcgyvqi9qywfg705Sr.*

Simple Addition #3

Add fatty fish rich in omega-3 fatty acids, like salmon, sardines, herring, anchovies, to your diet twice a week. Add additional sources of lean protein like chicken, fish, lean red meat, eggs, and beans. Prepare them in a healthy manner (baked, broiled, roasted, or grilled), using extra virgin olive oil instead of trans fats. Eliminate fried foods.

***HEALTH ALERT ***

Just because it's "healthy" doesn't mean it's okay.

Dietary guidance is essential for people taking blood thinners because what we think of as healthy foods such as spinach, kale and other greens will interfere with your clotting abilities if you are taking drugs to thin your blood. Your blood may, in fact, become too thin.

Speak with your healthcare provider before making dietary changes.

Foods or supplements containing vitamins K, E, or C may increase the risk of bleeding or interfere with medications like blood thinners or statins.

Grapefruit is known to interfere with medications for cholesterol, so be certain to consult your doctor, pharmacist, or dietitian before drinking or eating grapefruit if you are on a statin medication.

ALWAYS CHECK WITH YOUR HEALTH PROVIDER *BEFORE:*

- Taking Supplements
- Making dietary changes
- Beginning or stopping a medication

I know you've heard this, but...

There are thousands of diets and you must always consult with your physician, dietitian, or nutritionist before modifying your diet, especially if you're diabetic or taking blood thinners.

Keep it simple. Focus on eating fresh or frozen food with lots of color. Eat from the rainbow versus what is often the typical Standard American Diet (SAD) of white, beige, and brown. Get to know your local farmer at the market and eat seasonal, fresh, unprocessed food as much as possible.

TRY THE IDEA OF CROWDING OUT

Certified Wellness Coach Layton suggests the concept of *crowding out.* Simply put, this means adding more healthful organic foods to your diet to naturally crowd out the unhealthy foods. Eating more fresh and natural foods may increase your tastebuds' sensitivity. You may suddenly appreciate the sweetness of a perfect blueberry and gag at the weird taste of a blue Skittle.

Whatever dietary changes you make, Layton says, "Make it doable." She says, "I live by the 80-20 rule, which is: 80% of the time I eat textbook perfect foods that I know serve my body well, while

20% of the time I eat whatever I want. This mindset allows me to never feel deprived or 'on a diet'. Eating this way is not a diet, it's is a lifestyle, a way of living that will serve you for your long haul."

You already know that no two strokes are alike, but Layton says, "Each of us has differing dietary and nutritional needs, so there's no one pat answer for what each of us should or shouldn't eat." *Bio-individuality,*™ a term coined by the Institute for Integrative Nutrition suggests that no two people are alike and that each of us has unique food and lifestyle needs, so no single food philosophy or diet can yield the same results for everyone.

A person's lifestyle must be considered. Some people like to cook, others have no time or interest in cooking. Depending on what area of the country (or the world) you live in, the climate and season dictate what types of foods you eat. Our physical activity also plays a role in how we eat. Some do well eating meat, others are better off eating vegetarian diets. Some bodies can't handle gluten, while others don't have a problem with it. So, there is no one diet that serves all. If making dietary changes seems confusing and overwhelming, consider consulting a nutritionist or dietitian to create a workable and sustainable plan.

IT'S NOT ONLY ABOUT THE FOOD ON YOUR PLATE

Ms. Layton talks about "Primary Food," the foods that nurture and "feed" us but do not come on a plate. For example, our relationships, career, physical activity, and spiritual life play a huge role in how and what we eat. When these areas of our lives are fulfilling and gratifying, there is less likelihood that we will abuse our "secondary food" (the food that's *on* the plate).

"Sometimes we grab a carton of ice cream at 10pm, not because we are hungry, but because we're actually lonely." Food can satisfy a hungry stomach, but never a hungry heart. As Brooke Castillo, says in her book, *If I'm So Smart, Why Can't I Lose Weight?,* "If hunger isn't the problem, then food is not the solution." Becoming conscious of our feelings helps us create a healthier relationship with food.

CHOOSING HEALTHY FOODS IS AN ACT OF GRATITUDE AND SELF-LOVE

As Hippocrates once said, "Let food be thy medicine and medicine be thy food." Food is not our enemy; it's actually our medicine.

THE "MEDICINE" OF FOODS— VITAMINS FROM A TO E

- **Vitamin A:** Improves eyes and skin.
  Foods containing Vitamin A: Dark yellow fruits and vegetables (mango, papaya, carrots).
- **Vitamin B1** (*Thiamine*): Boosts mood, assists in positive mental attitude, helps keep body energized, may strengthen immune system.
  Foods containing Vitamin B1: Beef, beans, asparagus, oranges, oats, sunflower seeds, green peas.
- **Vitamin B3:** Helps boost good cholesterol.
  Foods containing B3: Tuna, chicken, turkey, salmon, peanuts, and brown rice.
- **Vitamin B6:** Protects against depression and memory loss.
  Foods containing B6: Fish, turkey and chicken, leafy greens, bananas, potatoes, and sunflower seeds.
- **Vitamin B12:** Essential for nerve health. Deficiencies lead to myelin sheath nerve exposure, causing neuropathy and pain.
  Foods containing Vitamin B12: Eggs, seafood, liver, cheese, leafy greens, milk, and red meat.
- **Vitamin C** (*Ascorbic acid*): An important antioxidant. Ascorbate is a regulator for over a dozen different neurochemicals and can reduce the risk of stroke.
  Foods containing Vitamin C: Citrus fruits, strawberries, and tomatoes provide immunity-boosting powers.
- **Vitamin D:** Helps regulate the immune and neuromuscular systems and builds healthy bones. Low levels of Vitamin D inhibit the ability to keep and form

new neural connections. Sunlight is needed to activate the body's natural production of this vitamin.

Foods containing Vitamin D: Fatty fish, mushrooms, and D-fortified foods. Because there are not many foods containing vitamin D naturally, it is often recommended that we take a vitamin D3 supplement.

- **Vitamin E:** Helps preserve brain function and protect against neural degeneration and may slow the rate of age-related cognitive decline.

  Foods containing Vitamin E: Wheat germ, nuts, sunflower seeds, avocado, leafy greens, sweet potato, and eggs.

Generally, you should obtain the bulk of your vitamins from a healthy and varied diet of natural foods, but three vitamins specific to stroke recovery can boost your body needs.

Remember, consult your physician before adding any supplements to your diet.

The Three Best Vitamins for Stroke Survivors

1) Fish oil is a concentrated and nearly perfect source of omega-3 fatty acids like EPA, DHA, and ALA. Fish oil is considered neuroprotective; that is, it protects the nervous system. Omega-3 fatty acids help the brain and heart in four ways:

- Lowers elevated triglyceride and LDL (bad) cholesterol levels.
- Promotes healthy brain function.
- Maintains healthy blood pressure.
- DHA and EPA may help reduce swelling in the brain after stroke.

  Aim for 250 to 500 mg of EPA and DHA daily.

2) B Vitamins help with nerve function and promote healthy HDL (good) cholesterol. Dr. Saposnik, a researcher on the Heart Outcomes Prevention Evaluation (HOPE) trials, suggests 2.5 mg of folic acid, 50 mg of vitamin B6, and 1 mg of vitamin B12 per day.

3) Coenzyme Q10 (or CoQ10) is a powerful antioxidant that protects brain cells from oxidative damage and helps generate energy in cells. This vitamin may be helpful for those taking statin-type cholesterol drugs, as it may prevent or treat the adverse effects of muscle pain and liver problems associated with these drugs.

HEALTHY GUT, HEALTHY BODY, HEALTHY MIND: WHEN BACTERIA IS A *GOOD* THING

Ilyse Wassermann Petter, MS, a nutritionist and the founder of *LettuceB,* a company opening organic, plant-based cafes and piloting plant-based children's lunch program, says of the gut-brain connection, "We are harboring ten times as many bacteria in our bodies than we are harboring human cells. There are trillions of microbes living on every surface of our bodies and most of these microbes are found in our intestines."

Although this may sound gross, it's not.

According to Wasserman Petter, "Studies show that 'good' bacteria or healthy bacteria reduce anxiety, lower our stress hormones like cortisol, and affect the neurotransmitter GABA (gamma-aminobutyric acid) that helps send messages between the brain and the nervous system. In essence, *good bacteria help our brains relax."*

Quite simply there is a direct link between the foods we put in our bodies and the health of our brains.

The body is a communicating organism, so it's not just the food we eat that affects our digestive system. Our state of mind also impacts our digestive system. Stress diverts blood from your gut and sends it to your limbs in preparation for fleeing or fighting. You know how your stomach feels when you're anxious, but you probably don't know that your anxious stress response causes your *digestion to be halted and impaired,* too. Chronic stress has long-term consequences on the digestion and absorption of food and the elimination of waste.

"We now know that these microbes living inside of our gut have a special relationship with the brain, communicating via the nervous system and interacting directly with our immune system. This tells us that in order to build a healthy immune system as well as a healthy nervous system, we must start with a healthy gut," says Wasserman Petter. "In addition to a clean diet (natural and unprocessed foods) and avoiding the inflammatory foods previously mentioned (sugar, hydrogenated fats) we must also consume the foods that *add probiotics and improve our gut flora.*"

Fermented foods such as coconut yogurt with active cultures, sauerkraut, kimchi, tempeh, kefir, and pickled vegetables all contain probiotics. In line with the principles this book espouses, Wasserman Petter says, "If you consume gut-healthy foods, eliminate inflammatory ones, and add the healthy mind practices of meditation and relaxation, you will go a long way in optimizing your health."

ESSENTIAL TAKEAWAYS

- Make dietary choices simple. Eat natural, unprocessed foods as much as possible. If it grows in the ground or comes off a tree it's better for you.
- Add more water. Aim to drink eight eight-ounce glasses a day.
- Eliminate inflammatory foods like sugar, refined carbohydrates, processed meat, and excessive alcohol, trans fats, and most oils. You can keep in "good" oils like extra virgin olive oil, unrefined coconut oil, flaxseed oil, and fish oil.
- Eliminate foods with preservatives, artificial sweeteners and artificial colors.
- Get the bulk of your vitamins from fresh food sources. Eat a nutrient-dense diet of food sources packed with vitamins, minerals, and enzymes.
- Consult your physician before taking any vitamin supplements, especially fish oil.

- Consult with your healthcare team *before* increasing your intake of dark leafy greens if you are taking blood thinners like warfarin or heparin. These healthy foods will naturally thin your blood so you may be at risk for increased bleeding.

- Ask your doctor about adding the three best vitamins for stroke recovery to your diet: Fish oil, B-Vitamin Complex, and Coenzyme Q10.

- Add gut-healthy, probiotic-rich, fermented foods to your diet for an improved gut-brain connection. Alternatively, take probiotic supplements.

- Let food be thy medicine. Healthy food choices are an act of gratitude and self-love.

BALANCING FATIGUE AGAINST PUSHING FOR PROGRESS (C&S)

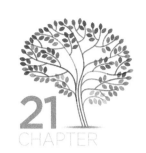

21
CHAPTER

*You are a human **being**, not a human doing.*

One of the most commonly heard questions/complaints from stroke survivors is, "Why am I so tired?" Approximately 40 to 70% of stroke survivors complain about fatigue. While post-stroke fatigue is often confused with "being tired," it's not necessarily the same thing and may not always be relieved with rest. This special brand of fatigue is called "neuro-fatigue."

Scientists have confirmed through PET scans that stroke survivors recruit more brain areas to perform normal activities than they did before their brain injury. Parts of the brain that previously showed little activity to perform a specific action now become actively involved through many extra bypass areas. In other words, it takes more brain energy to accomplish the same task.

A stroke is referred to as a cerebrovascular *accident,* and just like when there is an accident on the freeway, in order to get to your destination, you're going to have to get off and take the back roads. You can get there without using the highway, but it will take longer and be more tiring. This is what's happening in the stroke-recovering brain—it's taking more energy and time to complete tasks. Understandably, the more energy and time needed to complete tasks make one more tired.

Healing one's brain is a slow process. When an injury is "invisible," it's easy to forget the brain is still recovering from *edema* (swelling) and inflammation, while also painstakingly building new neural pathways.

Fatigue can be mental, physical, or a combination of both. It is a real, somewhat complicated, and regrettably inevitable part of stroke recovery. Much of your fatigue may be related to the energy-draining level of consciousness required to complete everyday tasks previously achieved at an automatic, unconscious level.

Chris talked about the fatigue he experienced simply walking into an unfamiliar location. "I have to think about every step. I have to tell myself to lift my foot on uneven surfaces. I have to remind myself to scan the environment. Literally, I talk myself through every step. Nothing is automatic, and it's exhausting. I often don't go places because it takes too much energy."

If you've never had an injury that interferes with walking, you don't *think* about walking. Only under the most extreme conditions, like an icy hill, unstable, rocky path, or a set of uneven steps navigated in the dark, do we give walking a second thought. But imagine if it was your daily experience. What if literally each step required conscious thought because your body no longer could rely on the normal feedback systems that allowed for automatic adjustments? Vision, sensory, motor systems, as well as *proprioception* (knowing where your body is in space) may be impaired, so that every step requires a conscious manual override.

After stroke virtually everything from eating to talking, to dressing, to walking is a form of new learning, and this requires an enormous amount of energy. When more than one task is attempted, such as walking and talking at the same time, the process can be exponentially draining. Add to this the expectations and judgements of others, along with a survivor's own self-recrimination, and you begin to see why some people don't feel like the effort of doing is worth the outcome. It seems monumental.

But not all fatigue is the same. Discovering its source can be helpful in managing and even eliminating it.

In medicine there's an expression: "When you hear hooves, look for horses, not zebras." Simply put, it means look for the simplest answers first. I encourage you to use the K.I.S.S. (Keep It Simple, Stupid) strategy for finding *solutions* to common problems.

What Else Could It Be? Sources of Fatigue:

- Pain
- Dehydration
- Medication
- Depression
- Poor sleep habits
- Sleep apnea
- Sensory overload: Too much visual, auditory, and/or kinesthetic stimulation
- Extra energy required for motor function and adaptive movement with weak or paralyzed muscles

Sensory overload can cause fatigue. Refer to this useful *Constant Therapy* guide called "Strategies for Reducing Sensory Overload in Social Settings": *blog.constanttherapy.com/18-tips-for-survivors-strategies-for-reducing-sensory-overload-in-social-settings*.

With this list of causes in mind, you can ask yourself questions to narrow down the source of the fatigue. Does pain keep your LO awake or drain them throughout the day? Pain medications can cause drowsiness, so balancing the two is often a challenge. This requires a thoughtful conversation with your doctor as well as experimentation with the dosage and timing of medications.

Is your LO getting enough sleep and water? You can't monitor what you don't measure. Is your LO getting 8 to 13 cups of water daily? Write it down as they go. Water is to a cell like a battery is to a flashlight. Cells require water to perform every function. Dehydration, even at a subclinical level, will show up as sluggishness, ineffectiveness, and weakness.

Do you and your LO have predictable sleep routines? What bedtime rituals does your LO have? How often do they wake up at night, and why?

Dr. Michael Breus, "The Sleep Doctor," a clinical psychologist with a specialty in sleep disorders and a member of the clinical advisory board for the Dr. Oz Show, says, "The number of hours of sleep needed are different for everyone. This can be based on age, genetics, medical history and medications." He's created a free Bedtime Calculator available on his website to help calculate what your needs are. *https://www.thesleepdoctor.com/how-to-sleep-better/sleep-calculator/*

His website also offers a free eBook, 10 Things Great Sleepers Do, as well as providing information on tested sleep aids and products, including a cannabis-based sleep aid.

Dr. Breus is a proponent of Cannabidiol (CBD). He says, "The cannabis plant is filled with hundreds of different compounds, several of which have been studied for decades for their therapeutic benefits. The cannabis compounds that have captured the most scientific interest are known as <u>cannabinoids</u>. Cannabinoids are now used in treatment for a broad—and growing—range of conditions and symptoms, from sleep and pain, to anxiety and inflammation, to Parkinson's disease and cancer."

He makes a very clear distinction that CBD is *not* the same as THC, the compound in the cannabis plant that has psychotropic effects and gets a person high. "Although CBD and THC are both found naturally in the cannabis plant, and are both made synthetically for medicinal use, CBD **does not** have any mind-altering effects. To the contrary: CBD appears to counteract the psychotropic effects of THC, which is the chemical compound in cannabis that delivers the "high" associated with marijuana. Just to reiterate, **CBD is a calming cannabinoid, with no 'high' or other mind altering properties."** Dr. Breus says, "CBD on its own has calming, anti-anxiety effects—one of the reasons why it's been identified as a useful supplement to treat insomnia and other sleep problems."

Dr. Breus adds, "Cannabidiol—or CBD—is a cannabinoid that's available in supplement form, and has a number of possible uses, including help with stress and anxiety, pain, and sleep problems. Unlike medical cannabis, CBD is legal in all 50 states.

Even if you live in a state where medical cannabis is currently not legal, you can still purchase and use CBD."

Many stroke survivors openly discuss their use of cannabis and CBD in the numerous online stroke support groups. I encourage stroke survivors do two things *before* using cannabis or CBD: 1) consult with their physicians and 2) find reputable and safe resources for these products.

ESTABLISHING GOOD SLEEP HABITS

Sleep helps your brain turn short-term memories into long-term memories. This process of consolidation works for muscle memory as well as general cognitive function.

In other words, sleep helps your brain remember how to do those movements and retain those thinking skills you've been practicing all day. I like to say sleep is like hitting the SAVE button on your computer after you've been working on a document.

The body thrives with regularity and routine, and establishing a consistent, predictable sleep routine is one of the best ways to do this.

If sleeplessness is the source of your LO's fatigue, here are 10 of the best practices for creating a healthy sleep routine:

1. Set the scene. Your bedroom should be dark and cool, at a temperature no higher than 70 degrees Fahrenheit.
2. Manage sound disturbances. Try white noise like a fan or noise machine.
3. Listen to hypnosis tapes or apps.
4. Trick your brain into a dream state. Simulate a REM (rapid eye movement) sleep state by looking straight up to your eyebrows and fixing your eyes on a spot. As your eyes flutter, know that you are simulating the REM state. You are literally telling your brain, by way of your body's actions, that you are dreaming, which is what you do during certain phases of the sleep cycle.

5. Do mental math. Start at 100 and subtract by 7s. (You might be asleep before 34.)
6. Consider *melatonin*, a natural sleep supplement that mimics a hormone responsible for regulating your natural wake and sleep cycles. *Remember to check with your doctor before taking any supplements.*
7. Sip hot milk or chamomile tea before bed.
8. Avoid disturbing news or TV, as well as blue light from tablets, computers, and phones at least an hour before bed.
9. Decrease pain by applying heat packs or warming blankets.
10. Use pillow props to help support a subluxated limb. Ask your doctor about magnesium supplements to help with muscle cramps.

Remember to check with your doctor before taking or stopping any vitamins, supplements, or medication

TO PUSH OR TO REST: THAT IS THE QUESTION

I am always asked, "How do you know when to push or when to rest?" The truth is, you don't always know, and inevitably you will get it wrong sometimes. The best way to determine the right balance is to check in frequently with self-assessments.

Use a 0 to 10 rating scale to judge your fatigue level. Think of your energy like a tank of gas in your car:

10 = A full tank of gas — Lots of energy

5 = A half-tank of gas — Moderate fatigue

0 = Gas tank is empty, call for a tow — Severe fatigue

In the beginning, with seemingly little expenditure of energy, your LO may quickly get to less than half a tank of gas or, in other words, be below a 5. They may need frequent mini-breaks to build up endurance.

The same is true for mental expenditures of energy. Every person will have a different tolerance level, and every day can be different, depending on how well they slept, ate, pooped, or worked the day before.

The real way to measure progress is to track it.

Keep a log, or use the companion journal to this book, *Hope After Stroke: My Recovery Journal*. It will help you and your LO see measurable progress and help guide you toward making adjustments as you move forward.

Rehab and recovery require the discipline of an Olympian. You have to show up, suit up, and engage in some daily acts of self-care *no matter what*. That's not to say rehab should feel like a Herculean effort. In fact, exercising your mind to see and believe in your recovery might be the only thing you do some days. On others it will be the warm-up activity before physical movement. Visualization is as important as movement. Practicing meditation and mindfulness will build cognitive endurance.

Your LO will have to learn when to push themselves and when to rest and trust that they will develop the self-awareness to be an accurate judge. Keep providing the rating scale to help your LO identify their energy level with a number. When attempting to help your LO notch up their endurance, if you feel as if you have rapport, you might ask, "Do you think you could do one more, go five minutes longer, or beat your record from yesterday?" Make the inquiry small enough that it seems doable, but substantial enough that it moves the needle forward.

Acknowledge any effort. Eventually your LO will learn to ask their own question in a self-coaching way, "Can I just _____?" See Chapter 23 Powering Your Goals with "Why" Fuel for more information.

POWER NAPS AND THE BENEFITS OF ALL THOSE *ZZZ*'S

Power naps lasting between 20 minutes and 1 hour can be the secret to supercharging your brain power. Survivors should try to take a midday rest not too close to an actual bedtime so as not to interfere with your longer night's sleep schedule. Researchers at the RIKEN-MIT Center for Neural Circuit Genetics say, "The sleeping brain must replay experiences like video clips before they are transformed from short-term into long-term memories." Sleep *prior* to learning helps prime the brain for the initial formation of memories, and sleep *after* learning helps cement that new information.

Sleep also removes the toxic proteins from your brain that have the potential to accelerate neurodegenerative diseases like Parkinson's and Alzheimer's. Sleep is the *only* time this protein buildup can be removed.

ESSENTIAL TAKEAWAYS

- Fatigue affects 40 to 70% of all stroke survivors.
- Mental and physical fatigue can have a variety of sources from the simple to the complex.
- Investigate and manage the sources of fatigue that are manageable, such as dehydration, pain, medications, sensory stimulation, nutrition, and regular sleep schedules.
- Optimize sleep strategies.
- Sleep is necessary to form and consolidate new memories and motor movements in order to turn them into long-term storage memory and automatic behaviors.
- Use a self-rating assessment to learn when to push and when to rest.
- Expect you will make mistakes. Learn from them and take a nap.

LET'S GET PHYSICAL: YEP, I'M TALKING SEX (C&S)

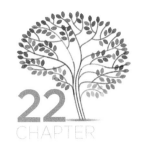

22
CHAPTER

The need for love and intimacy is a fundamental human need,
as primal as the need for food, water, and air.
~ Dean Ornish, M.D. ~

As long as we're in the bedroom… let's talk about sex. Sex is a virtually untouched topic of stroke recovery, but just because no one's talking about it, doesn't mean it's not on caregivers' and survivors' minds.

WHAT DO STROKE SURVIVORS WANT?

"Most stroke survivors are interested in sex and want more information about it," says Dr. Sara Palmer, a rehabilitation psychologist at Johns Hopkins University Department of Physical Rehabilitation, who researches and writes about sex and sexuality after stroke.

Dr. Palmer's research shows:

- Stroke survivors continue to have a sex drive.
- Sexuality is an essential part of a survivor's identity.
- Most survivors want to engage in some type of sex act whether they have a regular partner or are single.
- Most couples want to continue their intimate sexual relationship after a stroke.

Dr. Palmer says, "Sex is a basic human drive, such as hunger, and involves sexual function and sex acts. *Sexuality* is based on your feelings and values about sex, your sexual orientation and gender identity, and your self-expression and body image. Sex acts are included in sexuality, but they are not necessary to the expression of sexuality."

Sex and intimacy are wonderful healing tools and certainly contribute to a feeling of wholeness, but only at the *right* time and if both parties are willing and desirous. Chase and Annie are a perfect example of this.

Chase endured a long hospitalization as he recovered from a burst aneurysm that left him paralyzed on his right side and with hardly any usable speech. He and his wife, Annie, had been married for only five years when they were forced to be apart for over two months, including the month he spent in a semi-comatose state. It was emotionally difficult for both of them because they longed for each other like 20-year-old newlyweds, even though they were in their late 40s. Annie visited daily and when Chase finished his therapies, you could often find them cuddled together in his single hospital bed. Despite Chase's severely limited speech, Annie never felt like she couldn't communicate with him. "Even if he didn't have the words, I always understood him," she said. Despite his limited speech, his intelligence was obvious, and everyone on the rehab floor loved working with Chase. He was animated, had a good sense of humor, and was doggedly persistent in every therapy session.

During his hospitalization, doctors discovered Chase had yet another looming aneurysm, but before they could surgically "clip" the ballooning vessel to prevent another bleed, he had to heal from his initial surgery. Chase's wedding anniversary was nearing, and the doctors felt a home visit would be good for his emotional wellbeing. They believed his aneurysm didn't pose an imminent danger.

Chase was excited about his weekend reprieve from the hospital and eager to go home and finally have private time with Annie.

The following Monday morning we had our therapy session.

"Hi Chase! Was it great to be home?" I asked.

He lit up, and grinning from ear to ear, exclaimed with surprising fluency,

"I had a two-by-four hard-on!"

I don't know if I was more startled by his improved speech or by *what* he said, but I *actually fell* off my chair. Admittedly, it was not my most professional moment.

> *"Amazing!"* I said, fumbling to assemble picture cards and regain my composure. *"Maybe a little too much information, Chase, but I'm so glad you had a great weekend."*

Clearly sex was good for Chase's overall wellbeing *and* his speech fluency. Chase and Annie did what most people don't do because of fear or embarrassment; they simply asked their doctor the million-dollar question on everyone's mind: *Will my LO have another stroke during, or as a result of, having sex?*

Only your doctor can answer that question and advise you of the precautions and risks. However, it's good to know that during sex, one's breathing and heart rate acceleration are roughly equivalent to the levels seen after climbing two flights of stairs.

Dr. Heidi Moawad, a neurologist, and contributing health writer to the online site, *VeryWell Health*, writes, "Overall, it is quite unusual for someone to experience a stroke during sexual activity. In fact, it is rare for a stroke to be provoked by any immediate trigger. The vast majority of the time, a stroke is the result of a build-up of long-term health problems such as smoking, high blood pressure, elevated fat and cholesterol levels, poorly controlled diabetes, blood clotting abnormalities and heart disease.

However, there have been documented instances of a stroke occurring during or shortly after sexual activity. The case reports in the medical literature that describe stroke happening during or within 2 hours after sexual activity interestingly point to a higher likelihood of sex-related stroke in the context of extramarital relationships.

It has also been noted that extramarital sexual activity increases the risk of stroke-related death. Whether this is due to an increased stroke rate associated with emotional or psychological factors related to extramarital sexual activity, or to a reluctance to call for urgent medical attention is not clear."

For those with brain aneurysms the risks are somewhat different. A study by Dr. Monique H.M Vlak, a neurologist at the University Medical Center in Utrecht, the Netherlands found that having sex or drinking coffee could temporarily raise the risk of the aneurysm rupturing and causing a stroke; though the increased risk lasts for only about an hour after the activity.

Surprisingly, researchers found that coffee more than doubles the risk (for rupturing an aneurysm) versus sex. They found "drinking coffee raises aneurysm rupture risk by 10.6 percent, vigorous exercise increases the risk by 7.9 percent and nose-blowing by 5.4 percent. Meanwhile, sexual intercourse comes in at the lowest increased risk of 4.3 percent."

When I read that study I thought, *Skip coffee—have sex.* But of course consulting your physician is your best bet for understanding your risks and making appropriate adjustments.

The reality is not everyone is ready or eager to approach this phase of recovery. Just as every brain is uniquely different, so is every relationship. Sex is one of those issues couples are continually sorting out. If your sex life before stroke was challenged, it might be a bigger problem after stroke. Even before a stroke, one partner might have desired sex more than the other, and that disparity, when determining what's *satisfying,* can lead to even more stress and tension.

A caregiver's desire can be impacted and lessen for many reasons, including fatigue and the sudden shift in roles played in the relationship. The role of giving care is more parental and unsexy than being an equal partner, but sometimes surprising and unexpected outcomes occur.

David and Marissa had been married for over 20 years when David suffered a debilitating stroke that left him unable to return to his high-powered executive job. But what he lost in job satisfaction, he found in his relationship. Marissa said she and her husband grew closer because they spent more time together and they began to feel a deeper connection. She spoke wistfully about taking showers together, an indulgent pleasure they'd never had time for before. Marissa and David agreed their relationship was surprisingly enhanced after his stroke, mostly because they were willing to redefine what was important and to find ways to increase their intimacy.

If your sex life was previously satisfying, you can find ways to recover a gratifying and meaningful relationship if you're willing to explore, experiment, and expand your thinking. Open communication is best. If you haven't thought to ask these common questions, because of fear, shame, or guilt, know that they are normal. You might consider speaking with a psychologist trained in sexuality who can help validate your feelings and help you find resourceful solutions to the following questions:

- Will my partner be repelled by my altered appearance?
- What do I do if I am repelled by my partner's appearance?
- Will sex cause pain, especially if a person is suffering with spasticity?
- How can we communicate because of aphasia, apraxia, and/or dysarthria?
- How can we adjust our positioning for a paralyzed person?

INTIMACY PRECEDES INTERCOURSE

For many, intimacy precedes intercourse, and there are many ways to achieve intimacy without sex. Annie recommends "Flirting, kissing, hand-holding, and going on a date together to increase your level of fun, comfort, and bond with one another." What helped her in the later years after Chase had a second stroke and their sex life diminished was asking herself, "What am I trying to preserve?" For her it was "a deep connection and partnership with someone I loved," and she was always able to find ways to achieve that.

Finding ways to connect, even in the absence of sex, is important to the strength of relationships. Dr. Mitchell Tepper, a certified sexuality educator and counselor, says, "Contrary to popular belief, satisfying sex doesn't derive only from the genitals. Trust, safety, and connectedness are the pillars of deep intimacy."

Dr. Tepper should know; he suffered a spinal cord injury in a diving accident that left him paralyzed from the waist down. When no one could give him information about his future sexuality, except that he had less than a 10% chance of being able to father children, he dove into researching and dedicating his life's work to finding solutions for helping people with disabilities.

With a master's degree in public health from Yale and a Ph.D. in sexuality from the University of Pennsylvania, his mission was to end the silence around sexuality, disability, and other medically related conditions. He currently offers counseling, coaching, education, and a series of sex and paralysis videos aptly named Sexual Positions for Men and Women with Paralysis: Creativity, Adaptability, and a Sense of Humor. You can view the videos here (*www.drmitchelltepper. com/sex_and_paralysis_positions_for_women*) and here (*www. drmitchelltepper.com/sex_and_paralysis_positions_for_men*).

For more information, see Appendix Resources: Things that Make Life Easier. Look for the section on Sexual Health for a link to Dr. Tepper's website and information.

SOME SOLID SEX TIPS AND PRACTICAL CONSIDERATIONS FOR THE SURVIVOR

Timing, Props, and Positioning

If you want to bring your sexy back, don't look down, look up. Your brain is the most important sex organ you have. Anything that happens below the belt gets its jumpstart in your mind. Remember, our feelings create our thoughts, which direct our actions, which create our results. Visualizing, imagining, and using all of your senses to begin appreciating your own body sets the tone for you to appreciate your partner.

Kait Scalisi, MPH, a sex educator, writer, and consultant, says, "Think of appreciation as foreplay." Appreciating your partner with words or tender actions can be a huge turn on.

Experiment with *curiosity* instead of expectation. Sex takes energy, so consider *when* your energy is at its highest: is it in the morning, shortly after waking up, or in the afternoon after a rest?

Props like vibrators can help a survivor or caregiver if manual dexterity is impaired. The vibrator Ferticare is three and half times more powerful than a regular vibrator (useful when there is little or no sensation below the belt), and it requires a doctor's prescription. It's also pricey, around $600 to $700, but it's a very effective product used by spinal cord injured patients who have no volitional movement. It can help men ejaculate and may be used to aid in pregnancy. Medications like Viagra may also be options, but you must consult your physician to see if you are an appropriate candidate.

Nick Mahler, of Dallas Novelty Sex Toys, is a paralyzed man born with a rare autoimmune condition called fibrodysplasia ossificans progressiva (FOP) that slowly turns his muscles to bones, but that hasn't stopped Nick from having an active and enjoyable sex life with his wife of 17 years. He says he is committed to one goal: helping people with disabilities have orgasms.

When it comes to making sex toys for people with limited mobility, it really is all about getting creative. "We suggest our disabled customers use already existing toys in a different way," says Mahler. "Disabled sex toys are the same sex toys we sell to able-bodied customers. What makes them for disabled customers is knowing how to use them in a different way than an able-bodied customer." You can check out their props at *www.dallasnovelty.com*.

Kait Scalisi is a strong proponent of toys for women like the We-Vibe Touch, as well as G-spot toy Je Joue Uma and arousal oils like ON Arousal Oil, which she says brings blood flow to the vaginal area and make it easier to become aroused and achieve orgasm. Scalisi says, "Water-based lubes like Sliquid Organics are great for toys while silicone-based lubes like the one by Pjur are better for intercourse, oral sex and fingering. The amount of natural lubricant a woman produces is not indicative of her level of arousal as everything from stress to dehydration to medications can affect the body's ability to get wet." See the Appendix for a link to Scalisi' website and her list of resources.

Positioning is a matter of experimentation and using pillows. *Plenty of pillows.* You can use pillows to prop and protect your sassy (stroke-affected) side. Some positions that work are: (1) on your sides facing each other, with one partner's leg over the other; (2) on your sides facing in the same direction; (3) on your back with the more mobile person on top. If you take medication for spasticity, you might ask your doctor if it's safe to take an extra dose before having sex to keep your muscles relaxed. However, if you're male, the medication may interfere with having an erection and ejaculating, because, understandably, you can't achieve an erection with relaxed muscles.

Masturbation and Pleasuring Your Partner

Even though sex is considered a normal activity of daily living (ADL), it's unlikely your physical or occupational therapist will formulate a masturbation goal for you. Nonetheless, it's important to seek answers for questions related to masturbation and pleasuring your partner if you have the desire, but have limited hand or oral dexterity. Seek the advice of a specialist who is comfortable with and knowledgeable about achieving a satisfying sexual life in adaptive ways.

Birth Control and Pregnancy

Getting pregnant and preventing pregnancy carry extra risks for stroke survivors of childbearing age. It's important to talk to your doctor about the risks and precautions of both. Birth control pills are known to increase the possibility of blood clots, so discuss safer contraceptive alternatives that fit your lifestyle.

Incontinence

Incontinence after stroke is an incredibly common but troublesome problem that makes having sex slightly trickier. Let's face it, it's hard to relax and feel comfortable if you think you might spring a leak. But many stroke survivors overcome or manage incontinence with a few simple, common-sense strategies, including using the bathroom and limiting the amount of liquid you drink just before having sex, and avoiding positions that put too much pressure on your bladder. You can also feel more relaxed and confident if you protect your bed by using an incontinence pad, so if there is an accident, cleaning it up is simple.

Recovering Connection, Intimacy, and Love

Sex may be a human drive, but *love* is a human *need,* and it is present for the duration of our lives. Intimacy and love are possible even if you aren't having sex, but recovering intimacy takes time.

To do so, focus on connection and appreciation. Recognize that both partners are adjusting to major changes. Start simply and slowly, without expectation other than comfort and feeling good. Closeness and cuddling can be a starting point for exploration. You will likely have to experiment with positioning, even for cuddling, if there is paralysis or loss of feeling. Be willing and open to a sense of humor about any potential awkwardness, use of props, or unusualness of positions. Talk about what feels good and adjust and experiment accordingly. If both partners are open about their feelings and desires, intimacy can return.

GETTING HELP

The American Association of Sexuality Educators, Counselors and Therapists may be able to help you identify a therapist specially trained to help persons with disabilities. Send an email with the subject line "Referred by Stroke Connection Magazine" to aasect@ aasect.org, and ask if they can help you find a specialized therapist or counselor in your area. For general information, visit *www.*

aasect.org. Dr. Tepper is a certified sex educator and therapist and can be reached for personal coaching or consultation at *www. drmitchelltepper.com/contact*.

CONSIDER *ADAPTED* TANTRA YOGA: TRY THE HAND TO HEART POSE FOR CONNECTING

Tantra yoga is a style of yoga that focuses on the subtle energies within the body to enhance spiritual growth and physical wellbeing. While it is often associated with sexual acts, its foundation is based on the principal of intimacy and the act of connection. Traditional tantric poses may be challenging for a person with paralysis, but some poses, like the Hand to Heart pose are easily achieved. This yoga pose is aphasia-friendly, too, because no words are required for this communication connection. This simple but powerful pose can create great feelings of intimacy.

How to Do the Hand To Heart Pose

Stand or sit facing one another. Look into each other's eyes. Without speaking words, keep your connection with your eyes. Each of you place the palm of your hand over your partner's heart and feel each other's heartbeat. Next, focus on slow and harmonious breathing. Little by little, synchronize your breathing until you feel a calm connectedness. Take as long as you need to harmonize your breathing, and continue as long as you wish all while keeping your eyes gazing at one another. While this pose helps couples connect and communicate without words, if desired, upon completion, you may also take time to share what you felt and discovered.

ESSENTIAL TAKEAWAYS

- Sex is a human drive, but love is a human *need* present for the duration of our lives.
- Sexual desire for both caregivers and survivors may or may not lessen after stroke.

- Connection and intimacy, even in the absence of sex, are important to a relationship.
- Focus on connection and appreciation. Consider beginning slowly with cuddling and closeness.
- Experiment with props and positions.
- The brain is our most important sex organ. Use it to visualize and imagine with all your senses. Use appreciation of your partner as foreplay.
- Consider adapted tantra yoga for establishing connection and intimacy.
- Consult your physician regarding potential risks of sexual activity after stroke.
- Consult your physician regarding birth control and family planning after stroke.
- Resources including coaching, counseling, and education for sexual positions for people with paralysis appear in the Appendix. Look for the section on sexual health.

POWERING YOUR GOALS WITH "WHY" FUEL (C&S)

23
CHAPTER

Goals seem impossible only when you are not heading toward them.
~ Mike Hawkins ~

L et's get out of the bedroom and down to business. During the subacute phase of your recovery, rehabilitation is your primary job. Neurons are at their peak potential for rewiring, and neuroplasticity is the brain's mechanism for achieving those connections. It's time to use it or lose it.

The S.M.A.R.T. model of goal setting has been around for decades and it still holds up as a good foundation, but it's missing the "X" factor that takes goal setting to a new level. To make goals sustainable they need to *pull you toward them.* Too often goals are set with the *stick* approach instead of the *carrot,* and a goal that pushes rather than pulls is likely to be abandoned as soon as those inevitable obstacles show up.

WHAT'S THE S.M.A.R.T. MODEL OF GOAL SETTING?

It's one in which you make your goals:

- S: Specific
- M: Measurable
- A: Attainable
- R: Relevant
- T: Time Bound, meaning there is a date by which you plan to achieve the goal

So what's the missing "X" Factor?

It turns out the "X" factor is actually the question *Why*. Why is the most important question to ask when setting your goal. There are many, many ways you can achieve your goal, but knowing why keeps that inner desire stoked, propelling you to blast through challenges.

Remember Larry from Chapter 14: Preparing for Homecoming Before You Leave the Hospital? Larry left the hospital with a tracheostomy tube, an oxygen tank, a suction machine, and a walker. The hole in his throat allowed him to breathe, but prevented him from speaking, because the air came out of Larry's throat at the level below his vocal folds. In order to have sound when we speak, air must vibrate through our vocal folds.

Larry was a tough-talking, Harley-driving guy's guy who worked in the scrap metal business. His life revolved around two primary things: his work and his family. He was desperate to talk again because he felt isolated and disconnected from others. I knew his goal was to speak, but I wanted *him* to know *why and* what the *outcome* of his *why* would look like.

My questions frequently seem dumb. I watch people roll their eyes as if I were an idiot missing the most obvious thing, but I don't presume to know a person's why. So I asked Larry, "Why do you want to talk?"

He mouthed the words, "I want to tell people I care about them."

When he focused on his outcome, which was to communicate and connect, he could see there was more than one way to do that. He saw that he could write, he could text, he could email. In fact, when he wrote what he wanted to say, his written words were deeper and more profound than those he would've spoken had he been able to use his voice. Of course, he'd already been writing to communicate basic needs, but not in that deep way of intimacy that he longed for. When Larry connected to his "why" it was *his discovery* that made him recognize he had the power and control to achieve his goal. Larry achieved one of his outcomes even though his circumstances didn't change.

It was many more months of speech therapy and several surgeries later before he actually heard his own voice again, but his *whys* kept pulling him toward his goals. Larry eventually returned to work humbled by the applause, awe, and tears of joy from his entire staff when they heard him speak.

Even with a strong WHY, you sometimes might not feel like going for the gold.

Yeah, you've heard all the enthusiastic rah-rah, but the truth is sometimes you just don't *feel* like working on your goals. So now what?

Mel Robbins, one of the world's most influential motivational speakers, whose TEDX Talk garnered eight million views, developed *The Five-Second Rule.* Her simple method helps us crush the paralyzing *stuckness* that prevents us from achieving our goals, and it's based in science.

We already know the brain likes to conserve energy, so it tends to establish patterns. But not every pattern of behavior is resourceful or helpful. Remember, neuroplasticity can work for or against you. Habit patterns like procrastination can be interrupted. Once the pattern is interrupted, the prefrontal cortex can launch you into action and it only takes *five seconds.* That's right, there's a five-second window from the moment of your thought (*Gee, I should exercise*) to the moment of action. If you miss it, you'll remain inactivated.

SO, HOW DO YOU ACHIEVE ACTION?

Think of yourself like a rocket ready to launch. Seriously! Count it down loudly: *Five! Four! Three! Two! One!* As soon as you hit one, *take some action.* Stand up if you're sitting, or start to walk if you're standing. The more you repeatedly practice the act of moving from thought right into action, the more you will build a better habit pattern. Taking action will suddenly become a *"no-brainer."*

You can also use the simple phrase, *"Can I just___?"* Fill in the blank with one small, incremental action that will make you feel like you are moving in the direction of your intended outcome. Over time, tiny steps lead to big accomplishments.

Goal setting is driven by you. The goals you choose must be meaningful and matter to you.

Think about setting goals like this:

I want to do _____, so that I can _____.

Keep it *specific* and *avoid* the general answer: *So that I can be independent.*

Too often someone says, "My goals are to get back to normal." "My goal is to get back to work." "My goal is to walk again."

These are too general. Your brain needs a clear map of where to go and how to recognize when you've achieved that goal.

Even if your therapist gives you a specific goal (Do 10 leg lifts 3 times a day, 3 days a week), you have to know what that action is leading to. Ask why, with the curiosity of understanding how that action fits into the bigger picture. I'm doing 10 leg lifts so that I can _____. (Walk a block, for instance.)

Here are several examples of goals:

I want to use my hand so that I can sign checks for my business.

I want to use my hand so that I can cut my own meat.

I want to use my hand so that I can blow-dry my hair and put on makeup.

I want to use my hand so that I can masturbate. (*Yep, I said it, for the purpose of being authentic about people's desires, but you don't have to share every goal out loud.*)

I want to walk upstairs so that I can go to my daughter's home and play with my grandchildren.

I want to walk so that I can go shopping.

I want to walk so that I can travel and walk on cobblestones.

I want to walk so that I can get into my car, drive, and play golf.

I want to talk so that I can tell my wife and kids I love them.

I want to talk so that I can order my own food at a restaurant.

I want to talk so that I can tell a joke.

I want to talk so that I can dispute my bills.

It's obvious you want to use your arm, hands, and legs for every activity that defines total independence, but drilling down to those immediate **Specific** tasks enables you to **Measure** your progress in real ways.

The above examples show some of the *specific* reasons why you *want* to achieve your goals, and they are critical for getting clear and knowing what you are working toward. But there is a deeper level of why. Surprisingly that why is the same, regardless of the goal. It is simply this:

> *People believe that if they reach their goal,*
> *they will feel better.*

Let's go down this rabbit hole for a minute. Take any goal, even the broadest, most general: "I want to be independent."

Why? Because I want to feel like an adult again.

Why? Because I hate asking others to help me.

Why? Because being dependent makes me feel unworthy.

You believe that the condition of being independent will make you feel better, and undoubtedly it will, but the bad news is that might take a very long time.

So what's the good news? You don't have to *wait* to feel better. You don't have to wait and demand the conditions change in order for you to feel better.

You can actually feel better now. How?

By focusing on other things that you already feel good about. Initially that might be challenging, but you can always find *something* you appreciate. *When one is in a state of appreciation one feels better.* That is the purpose of the morning ritual (see Chapter 17: Managing

Your Mindset & Finding Meaning) to tune in and focus on what you appreciate.

The point is, if you practice feeling better now, in the present, you'll have already achieved a goal. When you feel good, you are more persistent. Persistence enables you to move through the stages of achieving the highest level of your goals.

Remember what we've said before: it's not the circumstances that control our outcomes, but how we respond to those circumstances.

This shifts the common belief, "I'll feel better *when*" (*fill in the blank—for example, I'll feel better when I can walk*) to "I'll feel better *then...*" *then* meaning I will first feel good and then approach the task. Feeling good, regardless of the conditions, is a master mindset that's achievable with practice. The more you practice feeling good, *the more you will want to do*. The more you want to do will translate into doing more, and the benefit of your repetitive practice will manifest in improved function.

MAKE GOALS ATTAINABLE

Make your S.M.A.R.T. goals attainable by breaking them into achievable pieces that will keep you inspired and your progress easy to see. Every physical action can be broken down into minute parts. For instance, if you're currently in a wheelchair and plan to walk as a goal, ask your therapist to break down the steps so that you can actively learn, practice, measure, and self-monitor your progress.

How do you write these goals?

Consider a speaking goal. Of course the big picture is you want to speak again in every situation under every condition, but this is grossly overwhelming and too big a leap from being aphasic and unable to say more than a few words.

Instead, pick a practical, functional goal: *I want to order food in a restaurant.*

How would you state it as a S.M.A.R.T. goal?

In our example, you might say, "On January 23, I'm independently ordering grilled salmon with a baked potato and salad at Francisco's Restaurant."

How would you accomplish this task?

Pick a specific restaurant and a specific dish to order. Practice the phrase, "I'd like _____ (the name of the dish)." Have someone videotape a close-up shot of just their mouth repeating the word or phrase over in a continuous, slow, and distinct loop. You will be able to watch and mimic the lip movements and language.

Put your mirror neurons to work. Mirror neurons aren't new to you. They're what's happening behind "contagious yawning." When we see someone yawn, we yawn. It's a little like monkey see, monkey do. Mirror neurons are cerebral motor neurons that fire in two ways: 1) when you move your own hands, feet, or mouth; 2) when you observe the actions performed by another individual. *Syncing up with another's movement teaches your brain to form a new pathway.*

Set a timer for five minutes of practice. Watch the video and practice speaking along with the person. Your mirror neurons are at work here. See Appendix Resources under Speech Therapy Apps: VAST for more information.

How Successful People Set Goals

Successful people practice the following behaviors when they set their goals. You should try them, too:

- Write down your goals.
- Plan how, when, and where you're going to achieve them.
- Speak your goal out loud.
- Engage all your senses.
- Visualize with closed eyes what it looks like to accomplish your goal.
- Utilize imagery and sensory experience. Practice feeling what it feels like. See, smell, and hear every element of your goal being accomplished.

Goals need to be **Relevant** and meaningful, so when working with a therapist make sure you are an active participant in establishing those goals. While it may be great for your motor dexterity to roll socks together, if you never did it before and don't intend to do that activity as part of your daily life, find something more meaningful that can achieve the outcome of the motor dexterity you need to develop.

Make your goals **Time-Based**. Knowing *when* you plan to achieve a goal keeps you motivated and diligent in practice. I've worked with many people who've had an event like a wedding to motivate them. They say, "My goal is to walk my daughter down the aisle" or "dance at my son's wedding." Pick a time, and if perchance you arrive at that date and you still haven't met your goal, acknowledge what you have accomplished, then refine and redefine the goal, and pick a new date. Dates are important. We have 365 days on our calendars, and not one of them says *someday*.

Practice your goals frequently and in tiny, incremental bits. Monitor them. Measure them. Don't wait for perfection to feel good; celebrate your practice and progress. Practice and progress, after all, are manifestations of success.

ESSENTIAL TAKEAWAYS

- Goals are driven by you. As such, they must be meaningful and matter to you.
- Make S.M.A.R.T. goals: Specific, Measurable, Attainable, Relevant, Time-Bound.
- Know your "Why." Goals driven by a strong why keep you motivated even when obstacles arise.
- Practice feeling good *before* and all along the way to achieving the goal. Shift your mindset from "I'll feel better when...", to "I'll feel better *then*."
- Use visualization and imagery to engage all of your senses to see, feel, and hear yourself accomplishing your goal.
- Celebrate your practice and progress. Practice and progress are manifestations of success.

PART 3

What Now?

Making it Work
When Everyone Leaves

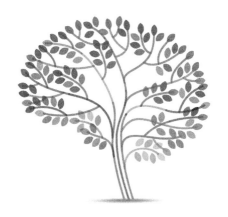

RESTORING ROUTINES (C&S)

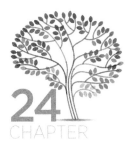

You are constantly invited to be what you are.
~ Ralph Waldo Emerson ~

The last day of home therapy and home healthcare can be a joyful milestone. The intrusions of therapists invading your personal space and driving your schedule are officially over. The silence and peace may be a welcome change or a terrifying prospect, or more likely a little of both.

Ready or not, the next level of self-regulation and independence comes with this transition. The upside is you've got your life back, the freedom to choose and make your own plans.

The downside is the enormous amount of self-discipline and organization required to maintain a daily program that keeps you and your loved one moving toward greater independence and recovery.

Hopefully you've followed the simple suggestions in Chapter 19: Getting on Autopilot. If you skimmed over that chapter, I encourage you go back and read it again. Establishing habits that become routine lead to successful self-regulation and greater independence.

You can start by planning what you'll do when everyone leaves.

There are four basic planning questions to consider:

- What will the survivor do?
- Where will the survivor go?
- How will the survivor get there?
- Who will be with the survivor?

WHAT WILL THE SURVIVOR DO?

Once again, the morning is the prime time to establish a baseline routine for your day. These "Power-Ups" increase mental stamina and enhance mood; they can be done in whichever order suits you:

- Practice gratitude
- Meditation
- Tapping
- Journaling
- Exercise

Hopefully you've already made this sequence of events a basic part of your routine. If you've repeated it often enough you will be reaping the benefits of how it energizes the body and mind and sets the tone for the day. But now what? You've got a whole day ahead of you. Time to start planning.

CREATE A SCHEDULE AROUND ANCHOR ACTIVITIES

Anchor activities are those that recur at the same time daily, weekly, or monthly. These are easy to plug into your calendar and build around. Start with exercise, or refer back to Chapter 19: Getting on Autopilot for suggestions from the Menu of Activities.

Your schedule should allow for downtime, rest, and relaxation. Rest can be an anchor activity. Continental Europeans plan a two-hour lunch and nap regimen as part of their lifestyle— Consider living *La Dolce Vita* (The Sweet Life).

The schedule should have enough flexibility and transition time to allow the survivor to move comfortably and competently throughout the day. They should feel the schedule has meaning and purpose, is desirable and achievable. If an overpacked schedule causes stress, it's time to eliminate some activities. Finding balance as a person gains endurance and independence is a constant and ever-changing work in progress.

WHERE WILL THE SURVIVOR GO?

Dive into your community. Your local library offers a wealth of activities and resources. They offer interesting speakers, a variety of classes, art activities, and of course a plethora of reading and listening materials all for free or nearly free. You can even ask your local library to order speech therapy materials to add to their reference section, enabling you access to free therapy videos. See Appendix Resources for Speech Therapy. In addition, libraries provide computers, internet access, movies, music, and a space that is public but quiet. Librarians are always willing to offer patrons assistance in finding just the right materials.

Brooke didn't think much about my proposed outing to her local library. She'd complained early on that reading was hard. Books couldn't hold her attention, and she'd lose the concept of what she was reading by the end of a paragraph. We began with simple articles with enlarged print and lots of white space between paragraphs to make it easier for her brain to process. She was skeptical about going to the library, but agreed.

Several months after our formal therapy ended, I contacted Brooke to see how she was doing on her own. Brooke had lots of exciting news. She'd gone back to work and was re-engaging in some of her most beloved activities, including water aerobics. I asked her what activities she felt were the most helpful that we'd accomplished in therapy. She said, "The library! I always bought books, but now I go to this quiet place and borrow them. I can also get them online, so I can even listen to them. My reading has improved tremendously, and since the library is nearby, I walk there. I exercise my brain and body, and I save money doing it."

She added, "The other surprising thing you helped me discover was my own backyard."

Brooke had a lush private backyard with a trellised canopy of flowering wisteria that overhung the patio. Clumps of white hydrangea lined the perimeter wall, and there were delightful surprises everywhere you looked—a glimpse of unusual blue and white glazed pottery, a rusted statuary, or a funky shell arrangement. She said she'd entertained there often, eating alfresco under the twinkling lights, but she'd always been "so busy being the hostess," that she never stopped to appreciate the serenity.

Brooke added a special relic to the backyard. Together with her OT, Brooke took an abandoned table she found at the curb and transformed it into an art piece by creating a new veneer, a tabletop of broken blue and white ceramic pieces. It became a trophy reminder of her stroke recovery, symbolizing that shattered bits can be reconfigured into something beautiful. Brooke says she often sits in this quiet space reading and appreciating the peace and beauty.

You can also consult your local community adult education groups and senior centers. Call your local city government offices to find information on special day programs in your community. Check with local hospitals for support groups resources and specialty programs offered.

Explore outpatient hospital or clinical therapy programs recommended by your doctor, PT, OT, or ST. Contact nearby universities to see if they offer low cost or sliding scale therapy services. These therapeutic services are performed by graduate students working on their master's degrees. The students are supervised by licensed and credentialed therapists who approve and monitor the therapy sessions.

Hospitals and research facilities often conduct trials and studies for new drugs or therapeutic treatments, and it's possible for survivors to become a part of a study. See the Appendix for a link to a website that offers opportunities to participate in clinical trial studies.

CLUBS AND ORGANIZATIONS

If your LO previously participated in a club or activity, encourage them to return with or without assistance. Sometimes, people are embarrassed, even ashamed or at least self-conscious, and reluctant to return to activities where they believe they will be pitied or in some way judged or shunned. Most often these self-limiting beliefs are the person's own feelings of diminished self-worth. Acknowledging those feelings and going anyway could strengthen your LO's self-esteem.

Toastmasters International is a great organization for a survivor who wants to improve their public speaking abilities. With the help of Toastmasters, two extraordinary survivors, Kate Adamson, the author of *Paralyzed but not Powerless,* and Valerie Greene, the author of *Conquering Stroke,* have become so competent at public speaking, they've become paid national speakers, sharing their stories of hope and recovery at large events.

You can search the internet for clubs in your area. Meetings are offered at various times and locations throughout the day and are sometimes based on a theme (Wine Tasters, Engineers, etc.). Visiting and participating in meetings is free. It's important to explore several clubs to find the best fit.

CAN YOUR LO USE A COMPUTER TO CONNECT ONLINE WITH OTHER STROKE SURVIVORS?

There are many services offering tele-therapy or online group support, which is so critical to recovery of the whole of wellbeing. See the Appendix for resources under Speech.

Does your LO have a skill they can teach other survivors?

The opportunities for global sharing over the internet with self-made movies on YouTube can provide a meaningful and purposeful activity for your LO as well as a genuine service for another survivor or caregiver. I've witnessed a man completely paralyzed on one side of his body demonstrate how to tie his shoelaces with one hand. That is YouTube-worthy. In fact, there are at least 13 YouTube videos I've seen on that very skill, and it's helped at least 2 other patients I've worked with.

Once you've established anchor activities, find two or three floater activities that can be plugged into a routine to make life interesting. Perhaps a visit to a museum, a park, or a botanical garden.

Activities that involve music or art and are typically thought of as right-brained activities can provide new levels of stimulation that are not language-based, but that still speak to the creative and intuitive centers of the brain. Many survivors discover new aptitudes, skills, and interests in art as a means of expression even using their nondominant hand.

Please know that any of these activities will be more tiring for your LO than for you. Yes, you may be doing the lifting of the wheelchair and helping them navigate the hallways of a museum, but the energy your LO needs to be alert and engaged in these highly sensory-stimulating environments is enormous. Check in with your LO. Help them learn to recognize their fatigue points before they crash and burn. Refer to Chapter 21: When to Rest: Balancing Fatigue against Pushing for Progress for guidance.

In the beginning, consider short outings lasting 30 minutes to an hour including transportation. Opt for locations nearby so you don't expend energy on the act of getting there. A simple car ride can be stressful and uncomfortable for a survivor. Preserve that energy for the activity. Always remember to bring your VIP parking pass (handicap placard).

Stroke survivors often talk about priorities in energy conservation. Knowing one's strengths and weaknesses and being able to assert one's needs is a high-level skill important for independence. If your LO can be left alone to sit in a spot safely, it allows you the chance to peruse another part of a museum or gallery while respecting your LO's need for a break. It is good for both of you to give each other a little space.

Brooke described how she simply wanted to shop alone and wander through her favorite resale shop without being "guarded or hounded." She didn't want to talk with her friends as they shopped; she just wanted the independence to wander at her own pace. When I took her on such an outing, I stood in the distance, allowing her the space to be independent. The faith and self-reliance she felt at this simple task made her feel normal. Feeling normal and getting your life back is a goal for everyone.

A WORD OF CAUTION

Not having a schedule or plan of action may lead to inactivity or dull, monotonous, TV-filled days that may in turn lead to depression. A plan of activities that wakes you up in the morning is important to fuel the most basic needs of human existence: connection, significance, growth, and contribution. Connection and purpose mean everything, and having a reason to get up in the morning and keep going is the difference between recovery and stagnation. Stagnation holds the strong potential for severe depression.

HOW WILL THE SURVIVOR GET THERE?

Most stroke survivors must wait a minimum of six months before being medically cleared to drive, if the possibility of driving is even a reasonable expectation for them. In the meantime, many survivors learn to take alternative, free, or low-cost transportation to get to doctor's appointments, outpatient therapy, gyms, and even malls and leisure activities.

Many cities provide local free or low-cost transportation. See if your city offers:

- Dial-A-Ride
- Access®
- Local, specialized busses for seniors and those with physical challenges. Each town is different. The requirements for use can be as simple as having a

physician's note and obtaining vouchers or as involved as going for a personal interview with Access® to determine a survivor's eligibility.

Transportation resources and services abound like never before whether you qualify as "handicapped" or not. Many high-functioning stroke survivors are able to use services like Uber and Lyft as long as the survivor can:

- Communicate the destination verbally and use a cell phone.
- Problem-solve.
- Ambulate independently, including getting in and out of a vehicle.

WHO WILL BE WITH THE SURVIVOR?

If you are the stroke survivor and have reached such a level of independence that you are safe to be alone at home or use transportation and attend outpatient therapy, a gym, a day program, or even a college, explore all of the options listed above and determine what means of transportation will be best.

If you are the primary caregiver and decide to remain as such, you may be eligible for payment through the state disability program for caregivers. It's important to consult with a social worker to learn the terms and conditions of that reimbursement.

Perhaps you (as a caregiver) have decided to return to work, but your LO still needs care at home. You may employ a part-time caregiver to help with meals and other needs. Get the help of a social worker and your rehab team to identify the survivor's immediate needs, knowing that everything always changes and will need reassessment down the line.

Sometimes a friend can be employed to be a helper; however, it's important to be *very explicit* about your expectations, as what seems obvious to you may not be to another person. Make sure you are both in agreement about the details of what, when, and how much you are willing to pay, and what is expected of them in return.

Communicating up front and regularly will preserve your relationships with friends. It's okay to suggest a trial period with an agreement among all people, including input from the survivor, such that at the end of the trial you will *all* evaluate if it's working and/or if changes are necessary.

A WORD ABOUT FRIENDSHIPS AND THE IMPACT OF STROKE

Jenna Schaeffer, M.S./CCC, a speech pathologist who now works with stroke survivors and people with traumatic brain injuries, changed her career path from Spanish literature and economics to become a speech pathologist after her father suffered a traumatic brain injury in a bicycle accident. Before Jenna ever became a speech pathologist, she was "just a daughter" who was instrumental in her father's recovery. Jenna knows the world of recovery from an insider's perspective. She says this about the nature of changing friendships.

"In my experience, changing friendships have a lot to do with *adjusting to a new you* and coping with a new identity. Friendships are usually based on shared interests—both physically and intellectually. My dad's friends were from work and sports. After his injury he was no longer able to participate in either activity. His friends didn't live particularly close, and there was no longer much of a reason to spend time together. Another factor in any friendship is personality. My dad's personality changed quite a bit following his injury, which impacted the shared friendships he and my mom had as a couple. Some really close friends were interested in learning more about the changes his injury caused and were willing to put forth the additional effort required to engage in a conversation with my dad. Those who were willing to learn, adjust, and make accommodations for my dad were the friends who stayed. Those who stuck around accepted that he was different. They accepted the new Jim without making comparisons to the old Jim.

Large masses of 'friends' (some of whom are more curious than anything else) are around during the immediate aftermath of a stroke. But the number of friends steadily declines as the reality of what the impact of the injury means becomes apparent. As devastating as it is to lose many friends during these experiences, I have learned to not resent those who leave. I have also learned that those who stay are the ones that you want to have around anyway. I would also highly recommend connecting with families who have been through similar situations through online forums, support groups, and finding new hobbies that are compatible with the new you. My dad is no longer able to bike ride, but he has recently found a new community playing pickleball."

A very real but often unexpected side effect of stroke may be a sense of loneliness and isolation for both survivors and caregivers. Caregivers may be particularly vulnerable to isolation because of the sheer demands placed on their time and the all-consuming nature of their responsibilities. Keeping friendships alive requires time, involvement, and even money to go out to lunch or attend an event. Caregivers often feel they don't have enough of any of those resources, and as a result their friendships may slip away. In addition, couple friendships may be impacted because of the survivor's communication challenges. It's necessary to educate friends and family members about aphasia and the best strategies for communicating with the survivor.

It's also important to seek out support groups where you will meet people who understand the complexities of stroke. While virtually no one *wants* to be a member of a group that identifies with an impairment, stroke support groups are the best place to learn about local resources and develop new and meaningful friendships.

Annie and Chase met many couples with shared interests in their support group. She said, "We were able to enjoy evenings in each other's homes, go to restaurants, and even travel together on cruises, which was really fun. It was easy being with these people because everyone understood the challenges and could relax."

Dr. Jeremy Nobel, a Harvard Medical School physician, public health researcher, and the founder of the **UnLonely Project**, shares a sobering fact researched by Julianne Holt-Lunstad, "Loneliness is as lethal as smoking 15 cigarettes a day." On the other side of that, however, he says, "Social connections are keys to happiness and health." Connection is a fundamental human need. Dr. Nobel is on a mission to lessen loneliness by bringing creative art expression into the lives of those most needing to connect. The **UnLonely Project** provides innovative programs, tools, and exercises to enable individuals and communities to make, share, and receive art to be less lonely. See Appendix Resources under Mental Health.

Like their LOs, caregivers should dive into the community. Consider an art or music class or explore a new and never-before-tried activity. Seek *respite help* for one to two hours a week for personal time that allows you to connect with existing or new friends. Time and consistency are needed for maintaining friendships.

If a survivor is capable and ready, they may consider part-time volunteer work in an area of interest. This can help build stamina and endurance, increase socialization, and feelings of contribution and purpose. Jenna's father, Jim, briefly volunteered in the community garden on days he wasn't at the gym or library, and it contributed to his sense of meaning and purpose.

The website *www.volunteermatch.org* offers numerous volunteer opportunities in multiple categories by simply inputting your zip code. The effort and time caregivers and survivors devote to expanding your social circles will improve the quality of your lives by increasing your feelings of connection.

ESSENTIAL TAKEAWAYS

- Establish a morning routine: meditation, gratitude, journaling, and exercise. These activities enhance language, memory, attention, and endurance, and cultivate a positive mental attitude.
- Create a flexible schedule with *anchor activities* that recur regularly.

- Live like a European: plan a two-hour lunch with a snooze.
- Discover your community resources: libraries, local centers, and clubs.
- Choose transportation options best suited to your LO's level of independence.
- Isolation and loneliness are ranked as high as smoking as risk factors for mortality.
- Friendships will naturally change. True friends remain. Branch out and embrace new social groups and find areas of interest in new activities. Seek support groups and online social opportunities.
- Capable survivors may consider volunteer work.
- Find programs to explore music, painting, crafts, writing, dancing, singing, and so on as a means of expression and connection.
- Caregivers should seek one to two hours of respite care daily or at least several times a week.

GETTING YOUR LIFE BACK (C&S)

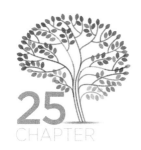

Don't look back, you're not going that way.
~ Mary Engelbreit ~

Ah, the chapter you've been waiting for....
Whenever I ask a stroke survivor, "What are your goals?" each and every one says, "I just want to get my life back." This is true for caregivers as well, although they might say, "I just want things to go back to what they were like before the stroke." The feelings of loss are so profound.

Alex, a member of a stroke support group, described his loss like this: "My stroke was like a thief. It robbed me of my ability to walk and talk and hold a job. It stole everything from me."

CAN YOU GET YOUR LIFE BACK?

Perhaps a better question to ask is, "Can I get a life worth living? Can I have a life that's meaningful and purposeful? Can I have a life in which I both contribute and grow? Can I have a life that is significant?"

What is it people really want to "get back"? Typically it's:

- Independence
- A feeling of worthiness and self-reliance
- Ease in getting around
- A sense of contribution and significance
- The ability to earn and provide

Everything comes down to independence, self-reliance, and a sense of self-esteem and worthiness, which all come down to one basic feeling: people simply want to feel good. Is it possible to recover those feelings even if the conditions of post-stroke life don't change? I'll let the Thrivers' stories answer that.

Howard suffered his first devastating stroke 18 years ago. He refers to the first part of his recovery as his "vegetable state." He was in a coma at the V.A. hospital for a month. After several months of hospitalization and a host of therapists who pushed him to achieve his highest level, he was ready to be discharged home in his wheelchair. The hospital social worker visited his home to assess his need and found a home care provider to make sure he'd be safe since he lived alone.

Howard waited at home for the arrival of the care provider, but when she didn't show up he refused to call and report it to the hospital. He feared they'd insist he return, and he was determined to live independently.

Instead Howard did his own version of therapy. As a former Army man, making his bed was as ingrained as brushing his teeth, but the challenge of changing his sheets and pillowcases with one hand became his therapy. He painstakingly worked one and a half hours on that task alone. This was his OT, PT, and ST task all in one. OT, because it worked his arms and hands; PT, because he mobilized around the bed. ST, because it was cognitively challenging to plan, sequence, and organize this task. Have you ever tried to put a pillowcase on a pillow using one hand?

This gave Howard the sense he was getting his life back and becoming independent. As his recovery progressed, he worked hard to obtain his driver's license. It took him one and a half years. He practiced on simulators and learned to drive with his left hand and foot. Throughout Howard's adult life, he had driven Harleys and sexy, sleek Corvettes, but according to him, his tricked-out accessible van that carries his motorized scooter is the "hottest" vehicle he's ever owned because it means his independence.

Daniel talked about getting his life back in a different way. He simply wanted a healthier life. He felt his stroke was a "wake-up" call alerting him to the things he was doing wrong. He looked at his diet and life stresses and decided to choose a different life that would enable him to give more, contribute more, and improve his wellbeing. He felt moved to share his wisdom and recovery with others especially in his stroke support group. He felt a sudden awareness of how loved he was and how important his relationships were, and he wanted to honor and appreciate them even more.

There is no one correct response to getting one's life back. Some physical and cognitive changes require complete reinventions that can at first seem impossible.

Sage suffered a stroke and *renal* (kidney) failure that put her at serious risk of dying. She was disoriented, incoherent, partially paralyzed, and very ill when I met her. At the writing of this book, she is still on the waiting list for a kidney transplant and has had four years of thrice-weekly dialysis treatments. When Sage examines how far *forward* she's come, though, she marvels at a couple of facts. During the most precarious emotional and physical time of her life, she homeschooled 2 children, one of whom was 10 years old and the other of whom graduated from *junior college* at age 17 and went on to Caltech on scholarship.

Sage recovered her ability to talk, write, and read, though she's not yet back to her desired level of articulateness. Long after her therapists left, she continued to challenge herself. She began blogging. Writing was difficult at first, but she improved both her motor skills and cognitive ones. Writing forced her brain to retrieve words, organize thoughts, formulate sentences, and spell. Blogging also served as a means of personal therapy—sharing her feelings as well as her insight and wisdom with others.

Once unsteady and dependent upon a walker, Sage relearned how to walk and now even rides a bicycle. Her hands that were initially too uncoordinated to feed herself are deftly knitting, crocheting, and quilting, turning out colorful caps, blankets, and quilts she donates to a battered women's shelter. How else does Sage contribute and find significance? She uses her talents as a former professional hairstylist to do charitable work. She says, "It thrills me when a client looks in the mirror and is excited by her new hairstyle."

Becoming independent was critical to Sage. Driving again enables her to get to the gym for an early morning swim before dialysis. She learned to swim at the age of 48. Why learn then? For over a year she had a catheter port in her chest for her dialysis. She was prohibited from getting in the water. She told herself, "Once this thing is out, I'm getting in the pool." Sage was afraid of the water because she didn't know how to swim. Still, she got in and said, "It felt great." She'd splash around practicing her "version of swimming."

One day a total stranger anonymously paid for Sage to have two swim lessons. Shortly thereafter, a friend at the gym paid for another lesson. She practiced what she'd learned in all three lessons and then watched YouTube instructional videos. Sage reports, "I'm finally swimming." Just recently another swimmer approached her suggesting she might want to compete, so she just added competitive swimming to her to-do list. Today, despite the extraordinary fatigue caused by her renal failure, she swims *twice a day*, continues to homeschool her daughter, and explore opportunities to speak and share her recovery.

Oh, one last thing, in case you have a spare kidney, Sage could really use it.

Did these people get their lives back? They'd say they stopped asking that question and asked a new question instead: "What can I do that makes my life meaningful?"

Do you ever get your life *back*? No one does. Life is never lived backward, but you can get a life full of significance, contribution, growth, and love if you decide to *live your life forward*. See Chapter 29: Forgiveness, Acceptance, & Reinvention for more stories of personal success and fulfilment.

ESSENTIAL TAKEAWAYS

- Instead of asking, "Can I get my life back?" consider asking: "Can I get a life worth living? Can I have a life that's meaningful and purposeful? Can I have a life in which I both contribute and grow? Can I have a life that is significant?"
- Whenever you need a boost, return to this chapter and read the personal stories and accounts of those who've constructed lives of meaning and significance.
- Life is not lived backward. *Life is lived forward.*

DRIVING & WORKING (C&S)

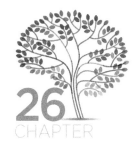

You will never feel truly satisfied by work until you are satisfied by life.
~ The Working Mom Manifesto, Heather Schuck ~

Nothing signifies a return to independence like being able to drive and go to work. Let's answer the first big question on everyone's mind: "Can stroke survivors drive?" The definitive answer is YES, *many do*. However, if you recall from Chapter 10: Answering Your Most Pressing "Why" Questions about Cognition/Memory, we touched on some of the concerns that need be considered before someone gets behind the wheel. Let's review.

Driving is one of the most complex tasks. It requires competency in three major areas.

- **Vision:** Approximately two-thirds of stroke survivors have some sort of visual impairment.
- **Cognitive Skills:** Attention, problem-solving, memory, reasoning, judgement, and the ability to be flexible in making quick decisions are all required in the act of driving.
- **Physical Movement:** Weakness, discoordination, spasticity, and paralysis are common effects of stroke.

Independent driving is only a benefit if the driver is safe.

GET A PROFESSIONAL OPINION

It's not always easy to tell if a survivor is capable of safe driving. More fights between caregivers and survivors can arise over differing opinions, and that can add great stress to an already stressed relationship. Not all doctors agree either, some release patients to drive without any assessment. However, most physiatrists are firm in telling survivors to wait a minimum of six months before driving. This is because vision is in a tremendous state of flux during this period. In fact, optometrists usually won't fill a new prescription for a stroke survivor before six months have passed, even though a person complains his glasses aren't "working."

Impaired depth perception, *visual field neglect* (missing half or parts of the peripheral vision field), and double vision are among the most dangerous visual impairments to driving. As the brain heals, vision changes, so it's best to consult with an optometrist to learn what to do during this actively changing condition. Sometimes, in the interim, purchasing drugstore "readers" can aid reading by enlarging print. "Readers," however, will not assist with double vision or field neglect. Occasionally a doctor may recommend eye-patching to lessen double vision. Persistent visual perceptual deficits may ultimately require visual motor training and/or prismatic glasses. Be sure to seek the services of a *neuro-optometrist* to aid with visual retraining.

Sometimes caregivers and survivors *test out* a person's skills in parking lots and on quiet streets, like they did when they first learned to drive. While that offers some insight into the survivor's driving capacity, it's important to remember that driving is far more complex than just knowing how to steer and put on the brakes.

I always recommend a professional assessment.

Who are the Professionals and What Do They Do?

An occupational therapist (OT) or a certified driver rehabilitation specialist is licensed to make assessments of all the skills needed to qualify your LO as a safe driver. You will need a *prescription* from your physician requesting OT services to assess driving skills. The diagnosis should say something about the type of stroke or could simply state "CVA (cerebrovascular accident)." The actual prescription should say, "Assess driving skill competency."

OT evaluations include testing for awareness of:

- Road signs and speed limits

- Visual scanning, depth perception, the ability to physically adapt and move to see obstructions, such as turning around when backing up
- Safety awareness of seat belts, lights, adjustment of mirrors, and windshield wipers
- Cognitive skills including attention, memory, following directions, impulse control, and problem-solving
- Physical road tests on both surface streets and highways. OT and driving specialists have specially-equipped vehicles with passenger controls to assure safe testing conditions.

The fee for this service is usually between $400 and $600, and although it's not covered by insurance, it is well worth the peace of mind for everyone involved. If a survivor does not pass the test, the OT will identify the areas of need and propose a course of treatment in a written and verbal report.

Consult your local DMV for services they may provide to aid stroke survivors in recovering the ability to drive.

"Pimp Your Ride" – Errr, I *Mean,* Adapt Your Car

There are many ways around physical limitations. An OT or physical therapist can recommend possible adaptations that will make driving easier. See the Appendix for resources listed under Driving.

Some examples of car adaptations are:

- **Spinner wheels**, which attach to your steering wheel for one-handed steering
- **Left-foot accelerators**, for those with right-side impairments
- **Swivel seats** that help you get in and out of the car

RETURNING TO WORK AND FINDING PURPOSE

Work is so integral to a person's identity and self-esteem that when the option to work seems as if it's been snatched away, a survivor can feel more than just the fear of financial loss; they may feel a loss of their humanness and self-worth.

Survivors are eager to return to work because they associate it with being productive and "normal," a sure sign of recovery. Work offers the opportunity for connection and the social exchange so vital to our wellbeing. It allows a person to feel a sense of contribution and significance that they are a valued member of a team, organization, or society in general. Work gives us a sense of purpose, belonging, and certainty that meets all of our basic human needs.

The pressure of mounting bills and the fear of how one will continue to live and support one's self and their family may prompt an urgent *need* to return to work before one is really capable. Work is, in fact, therapeutic for survivors and ideally an end goal of recovery, but it's important not to rush into it. Going back too soon can have terrible repercussions.

Dr. Matthew Fink, chairman of neurology at Weill Cornell Medicine and neurologist-in-chief at New York-Presbyterian Hospital, says, "When you go back to work, you want to be able to meet the demands of your job. If you go back too soon and don't perform well, it can reflect badly on your performance and cause problems with your employer, which can elevate your stress levels. Additional stress would be bad for your recovery. Also, if you return to work before you can perform well, you run the risk of losing your job, which would add more stress."

Ironically you may prematurely bring about the very thing you fear, losing your job, by returning to work too soon.

In my experience, I've seen greater scrutiny of performance with stroke survivors and those with traumatic brain injuries when they return to the workplace. Small mistakes that are overlooked all the time in the workplace, such as misspelled words, typos, or mix-ups in dates and times, are viewed differently when a known brain injury exists. You have a right to your medical privacy.

I always encourage limiting the information exchange with your employers until you have a clearer idea of your level of overall function and your longer-term intentions.

GET HELP FROM A SOCIAL WORKER

Social workers are your allies, and you will want them on your recovery team. Aside from helping survivors and caregivers deal with the emotional impact of a disability, they are experts in the intricacies of Social Security Disability Insurance (SSDI) and Supplemental Security Income (SSI). Government programs have *lots* of paperwork, and social workers can assist in filling out and filing the necessary documents to obtain disability payments while the survivor is not working.

While many stroke survivors do return to work, statistics show that stroke is the leading cause of long-term disability. This is a tough and sobering statistic.

Can a survivor return to work? Yes, depending on their level of function. Those with higher cognitive function, even in the presence of physical impairments, are more likely candidates to resume work, even if it's not working at one's previous job or even within the same industry. One of the hardest and most unexpected challenges is *how long it may take* to return to work. There are no hard and fast answers about the length of time it takes for someone to recover enough capacity to return to work. There are many variables and options to consider, so it's best to engage your team of professionals—the OT, PT, ST, and social worker—as well as your employer to ask questions and assess the who, what, when, where, and how of returning to work. Again, note that it may be best to contact your employer via your rehab team or caregiver, or to keep contact over the phone at first so that nothing damaging is in writing.

While you may not be able to return to your prior job after your stroke, there are services that can help you find *new* work that aligns with your experience, abilities, and interests. Allsup Employment

Services, Inc. (AESI) is a national network that provides free services such as:

- Career planning
- Work incentive/benefits counseling
- Resume building/interview preparation
- Job search/job placement assistance
- Ongoing support once employment is obtained

In an online article about returning to work, the National Stroke Association discusses the "Ticket to Work Program." The ultimate goal of this free program is to provide support that reduces a person's dependence on disability benefits and helps participants earn more income than their benefits alone can provide. Use this link for more information: *www.stroke.org/stroke-resources/ resource-library/ticket-work-program-information*.

I'll close out this chapter by sharing William's and Craig's stories. I hope they inspire you as you move forward in your recovery.

William was a dignified man whose crisp, starched shirts were only one aspect of his meticulous demeanor. He held a prestigious and high-level administrative position at a university. William's stroke left him struggling with spasticity in his right arm and leg. He had poor breath support that resulted in strangled-sounding speech, and he spoke so quietly he was barely audible. Over the course of eight months, William regained enough capacity to do everything he needed to return to work on a part-time basis with accommodations. He was able to drive, park, and walk the distance required from the VIP (handicapped) parking to the elevator to reach his office. He developed enough breath support for speaking, and his vocal volume was loud enough to participate in phone conferences and round table meetings. He was also able to verbally delegate jobs to various assistants.

William recovered enough motor function to successfully operate his computer, send emails and engage in written documentation necessary to his job. On multiple trial runs, with assistance from the OT and PT, William practiced walking from the parking lot, managing the doors while wearing a backpack and pushing a walker. He practiced accessing the bathrooms independently and exiting the building down the stairs, on his rear end, in case of an emergency if the elevators weren't functioning. He requested and received several accommodations from his employer.

First, he returned on a part-time basis, three days a week, for four hours a day. In addition, he obtained a couch for his office, where he could rest as needed; an adapted mouse for ease in working with his computer; and a voice amplifier on his phone. On his "off" days and sometimes after work, William continued with outpatient physical therapy. He was the only one in the PT gym in a starched white shirt.

From the first day I met Craig, he made it clear he wanted to return to work as a criminal attorney, where for 36 years, he had worked with the public defender's office on high-profile murder cases, the kind of cases that required the sharpest, most discerning intellect, reasoning, and memory skills.

Craig had a stellar legal mind. He was the attorney on 160 felony trials during his impeccable career of service. His stroke didn't impair his intellect. His mind was still keen, but he had severe Wernicke's aphasia. His type of aphasia allowed him to speak with relative ease and his voice and articulation sounded normal, but if you listened to the content of his speech, he didn't make much sense. He made up words (*neologisms*) and had no awareness that his "word salad" speech was mostly incomprehensible. It infuriated him that his wife couldn't understand him.

Craig also had severe visual acuity and perceptual impairments and couldn't read. Reading was crucial to his work. As if those weren't enough challenges, he had a heart valve that emergently needed replacement. He and his family feared the possibility of another stroke or complications that might arise during surgery.

Craig wanted to work. He wanted to reach his full pension level so that he could retire at 65. He was 60.

To do this, Craig was willing to give up the high-profile murder cases and return to the work he'd done years before as a junior-level attorney, consulting prisoners in jails to arrange plea bargains for minor offenses. His procedural memory for interviewing people was intact. In our sessions, he devoted hours of practice to asking questions and writing the responses during simulated conversations a prisoner might have with him. He became an expert at using strategies to get his clients to also do the writing for him.

Craig accepted the fact that right after his stroke he had *no* ability to read. His acceptance spurred him to earnestly begin at the beginning. He didn't allow his pride to interfere with his success. With diligent practice he made it to a kindergarten reading level. He persisted in reading books until he progressed to a third-grade level. We'd discuss the story, then he'd summarize it by recording himself on audio. As Craig listened to himself, he increased his awareness and self-monitoring of his speech.

With encouragement and direction Craig enrolled in a local college with a specialized program for people who'd suffered brain injuries. He spent another six months relearning computer skills, improving verbal communication, reading, and writing. Craig returned to work just as he'd planned within a year of his stroke and successful heart surgery. He's on track to retire at his full pension in 2020.

ESSENTIAL TAKEAWAYS

- Driving is a complex task. Most physiatrists insist on waiting six months before releasing a survivor to drive. Vision, cognition, and physical skill must be functionally competent before you can get behind the wheel.
- Seek the services of a neuro-optometrist to aid in recovering peripheral vision and improved depth perception.
- Occupational therapists can assess a person's competency for driving.

- Cars may be adapted for special needs to allow independence.
- Returning to work is a major goal of recovery.
- Stroke is the leading cause of long-term disability.
- Don't rush back to work. Take time to recover. Prevent job loss by recovering skills and stamina before returning to work.
- Limit interactions with employers during recovery. Avoid written correspondence.
- Consult with your social worker for help with Social Security Disability Insurance (SSDI) and Supplemental Security Income (SSI).
- Utilize social workers for coping with the emotional impact of a disability.
- Seek the services of vocational rehabilitation programs to prepare you to return to work.
- Engage your team (OT, PT, ST, and social worker) and employer to determine options for returning to work.

SOME DAYS ARE CRAPPY (C&S)

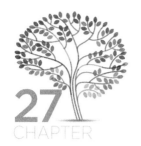

I could tell it was going to be a terrible, horrible, no good, very bad day.
**~ Alexander and the Terrible, Horrible,
No Good, Very Bad Day, Judith Viorst ~**

Let's get real. Rehab is not always a gloriously orchestrated movie-worthy hero's journey. (Oh, you already knew that!) There are really, really hard days, depressing days, and days when exhaustion, frustration, and despair seem to lead the way without letting up.

Yes, some days are crappy. Really, really crappy. And some days are not—like those constipated days when you only *wished* they were crappy.

Wait… Didn't I tell you in Chapter 5: Change Your Language, Shape Your Life that our language creates our reality? And now I'm saying, "Some days are crappy"?! Yes, because it *is* important to feel feelings, even the strong negative ones, from time to time.

It might seem like a contradiction to say this because my entire premise is about our thoughts, but our feelings do warrant our attention, curiosity, and compassion. Note here that attention is different than indulgence.

Attention means, "Let me hear you, know you, understand you, learn from you." Indulgence means, "Let me wallow in this feeling. Let me feel stuck. Let me feel powerless and sad." Feeling into the depths of your emotion can be liberating. No one has ever died of a feeling, but those who repress their feelings often have strokes and heart attacks.

I'M AFRAID IF I START CRYING, I WON'T BE ABLE TO STOP

Some people are so afraid to grieve or cry, fearing it will be a faucet that won't turn off, that it will provoke a condition of sadness from which they won't recover. This is a typical yet unfounded fear. There is a distinct difference between feeling appropriately sad and clinical depression.

Please contact your doctor if your LO's sadness or your own sadness is so persistent and pervasive that it interferes with and limits your engagement in daily activities. Only your physician can diagnose true clinical depression and help you make choices about how to manage or improve your situation.

Most often the "Crappy Day Syndrome" has to do with fatigue, resistance to what is or is not happening, and frustration. As you look for evidence of everything that is wrong, awful, and not working, you will find evidence and further confirm the so-called truth about your biggest fear: *I will never get better.* This pattern of thinking inevitably leads to feeling crappy. It makes sense that if you get on the train going to hell, it's going to be hot and awful when you get there.

What's the outcome you want? If you truly want to get better, you have to realize that you are on the wrong train of thought. Get off and take a detour.

TAKE A DETOUR: THE FIVE-MINUTE PITY PARTY

You can't deny a thought that's in your head. If you're told to *not* think about something, that's the first thing that pops in your head. Instead of stuffing the feelings and saying you won't think about them, allow yourself a Five-Minute Pity Party.

Yes, really. Set a timer for five minutes and wail, complain, and rant about every wrong thing in your life. Ask your internal self what it really wants. When the timer goes off, acknowledge your thoughts and thank them for sharing. Respectfully ask, "What do I want to feel now?"

If we examine what we *want* and explore it deeply enough, we'll discover that no matter what that *"want"* is, whether it's walking independently, a pile of money, or a loving relationship, *we believe it's the attainment of that desire that will make us feel good.*

But here's the thing: not only can we *feel good before* we get the thing we want, we *must feel good* in order to get that thing.

Ask: "What would I have to think *in order to feel good*, or at least better?"

If the answer to the question "What do I want to feel?" is, "I want to feel better," then start with Bridge Thinking. "Bridge Thinking" is a concept by Brooke Castillo, a life coach who teaches a course on *How to Feel Better.* Bridge thinking is what allows you to go from one diametrically opposed thought to its opposite.

For example, if the thought is, "I will never walk, I am paralyzed," then it's too great a leap to think or affirm, "I will run tomorrow."

You could instead begin like this:

I am paralyzed.

I can't walk, now.

I don't know if I will ever walk.

I can't walk *yet*, but I know some people recover.

I like the idea of recovering.

I like the idea of thinking I can walk.

It scares me to think I can't walk.

Thinking that thought makes it harder to try.

I wonder what thoughts make it easier to try.

I like the idea of believing I could walk.

I like the idea of believing I could stand.

Just thinking about standing makes me feel good.

When I feel good, I feel like trying.

When I try, I am more likely to make progress.

I wonder what it's like to try for just one second.

Can I just try standing for a second?

I will stand and count.

My goal is to count to three while standing.

If you're already in a revved-up state of crappy thinking, though, rest might be the best thing for you. You can halt the momentum of thought with a glass of water and a nap.

This act of going deep can be exhausting. Follow it up with a good rest.

****NOTE TO CAREGIVERS****

Getting some distance from your LO during this state or afterwards is a way for you to protect your energetic boundary. It may feel awful to watch someone you love suffer without having the ability to fix or change it.

You may be supportive, you may even offer tough love, but you also need to care for yourself. You are at the helm of it all, and you are the only one responsible for caring for yourself. You can't fix your LO because they are not broken. They are going through a difficult time.

While you may not think there is anyone else who can help, you have to be willing to expand your thinking.

Plant the question, "Who else can be a resource for me to enable me to rest?" in your mind, and write down the answers. Paid and unpaid help may be available. A neighbor, a friend, a family member, a church group, or a member from an affiliated club might come to your aid. Perhaps your LO is even safe to be left alone for 5, 10, 20 minutes, or a half-hour while you walk around the block, go to a different room, step outside, or even leave the house.

That said, your LO must always have access to a phone or an exit if they are left alone. Based on your LO's judgement and impulsivity, you must know the conditions under which they could be safely left unattended. Common misjudgments of a

---

survivor's level of self-regulation, impulsivity, and safety can have devastating consequences.

In general, never leave your LO alone if you believe they may injure themselves or be unsafe due to severe depression, impulsivity, poor judgment, decreased memory, or poor motor skills. This is especially true for activities such as showering and cooking, or if you believe they might potentially attempt to drive, or, like Thom, operate a chainsaw and then climb a ladder.

THIS, TOO, SHALL PASS

You don't have to be religious to understand the validity of this statement. Every day changes, every hour changes, every minute and every second changes. We only feel hopeless when we believe that nothing is changing.

Resetting and rebooting after a "crappy day," knowing that this, too, shall pass can bring a little relief. Do whatever (brain-supportive vs. brain-destructive) thing you need to do to facilitate a lessening of stress.

Here are some stress reducers I recommend:

- Tapping
- Deep breathing
- Singing
- Meditation
- A hot shower
- A nap
- A no-stress mental game like Flower Cells© on a tablet
- Classical music
- Journal writing
- Physical activity
- Watching videos of babies laughing
- Petting an animal

- Smelling lavender essential oils
- Watching videos of baby animals

A Word of Caution

Many people wonder about drinking alcohol or using recreational drugs to lessen stress.

First and foremost, always consult your doctor and be truthful about your intent so that as a team, you and your physician can understand the benefits, risks, and possible interactions with other medications of your "drug of choice." I offer neither moral nor medical advice about that decision, but I will offer a few facts.

Alcohol is a depressant. Pure and simple. It is a drug that may interact with other drugs, most notably antidepressants. What is the effect of alcohol on the brain?

Alcohol affects the part of your brain that controls speech, movement, and memory. In excess, it also may impact your judgment. If a survivor's motor functions are already impaired, adding alcohol will likely exacerbate motor and cognitive difficulties, including slurred speech, diminished balance, trouble walking, and difficulty thinking or performing divided attention tasks like walking and talking at the same time. Consult your physician before self-medicating, and try to find a healthy way to cope with the crappy days.

ESSENTIAL TAKEAWAYS

- Some days are crappy. Fatigue makes everything worse.
- Practice the phrase: "This, too, shall pass."
- Have a five-minute pity party and practice Bridge Thinking to tune your brain into thoughts that feel better.
- Choose brain-supportive stress reducers (see the list above for ideas).
- Caregivers need to get distance and support themselves.
- Naps are good for everyone.

PLOWING THROUGH PLATEAUS (C&S)

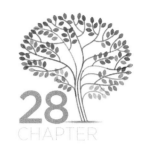

Just keep swimming.
~ Dory from Finding Nemo ~

You already know that the period of spontaneous recovery, that is, recovery without effort, occurs in the first three months after stroke. During that subacute stage of recovery, progress occurs more rapidly. The billions of neurons that were stunned come alive, and the brain is swimming in an almost magical protein called *brain-derived neurotrophic factor* (BDNF). This same protein is present at birth and is also released right after a brain injury. BDNF enables the brain to massively and rapidly wire neural connections.

In the next phase of recovery, called the Chronic Phase, the rate of progress is not as rapid. I'd personally like to rename this the "Make Your Life Matter" Phase, but at any rate, it lasts from three months post-stroke throughout the rest of your life. Many doctors tell their patients, "Whatever you've got now is *as good as it's going to get,*" but that's simply not the case. More survivors than not disprove that piece of information. It's a limiting thought to plant in the mind of survivors and caregivers because it falsely conveys that the survivor is at the end of recovery. Just like any ride that comes to an end, people get off. Getting off the ride of recovery is the only definitive thing that halts progress.

It's safe to say that as long as one is still alive, the potential for growth exists.

Reaching an *apparent plateau* may lead to an erroneous conclusion that no further progress can be made. This is a dangerous assumption because it can cause the survivor's disengagement. If one disengages from the process of recovery and thinks no further progress can be made, the inevitable outcome of learned nonuse or dis-use is a very real threat and the saboteur of future progress.

Simply put, when you think it's over, it is the start of it *being* over. Why?

Let's remember that our thoughts create our feelings, which direct our actions, which ultimately create our results.

Why bother? Why make the effort? become the survivor's primary thoughts when they think they've reached the plateau of "it's as good as it's going to get."

Plateaus happen when it gets much harder to see the evidence of progress. This flattening out of progress is what defines a plateau.

If you or your LO feel as if they've hit a plateau, here are several things to consider.

First, recognize it. Acknowledge it. Don't rush to fix it or change it. Be with the thought and curiously ask, "What else could it mean?" There are so many feelings that accompany the thought, "I've hit a plateau" that, before you can address and redefine a new goal, you must see what else might be holding you back.

Fear, anger, and sadness are real emotions connected with the thoughts, "I am not making any progress, or as much progress as I want, or fast enough progress." These thoughts create feelings that ironically undermine future progress.

When you are willing to recognize and examine the thought and feeling, "I've hit a plateau," things can shift. Plateaus may simply mean it's time to change a strategy or therapeutic modality. When something stops working or being effective, whether it's a business tactic, a shampoo, or a food that makes your dog go wild, it simply means it's time to **change it up** not time to give up!

The truth is we are constantly changing, either moving forward or declining, and even if you're simply holding the line against further decline, this should be viewed as progress. Maintenance is progress.

When you recognize and acknowledge the feeling of a plateau, it is an opportunity to Tap on all those feelings and see what's up. **To learn how to tap and what the tapping points are refer to this beginner video:** *www.youtube.com/watch?v=pAclBdj20ZU.*

SCRIPT FOR TAPPING

Click on this downloadable link to the Tapping Points Chart to follow along with the abbreviations below. <u>The link also appears in the Appendix.</u>

Meridian Points for Tapping
https://bit.ly/2GWIiw8

Start by tapping on the karate chop (KC) position and repeat the first phrase three times.

KC: Even though I'm certain I've hit a plateau and I am not getting better,

I still want to love and accept myself.

KC: Even though I'm sure I've hit a plateau and I'm afraid I'll never get better, I still want to love and accept myself.

KC: Even though I'm so angry, so sad, and so frustrated that I'm not making progress, I want to be open to loving and accepting myself, but I can't.

Eyebrow (EB): This fear I'm not making progress

Side of Eye (SOE): This fear I'll never get better

Under Eye (UE): This fear and sadness

Under Nose (UN): I'm stuck like this forever

Chin: This hopelessness and fear

Collarbone (CB): I'm so scared

Underarm (UA): I'm so sad

Top of Head (TOH): I'm so angry

EB: I work so hard

SOE: Not getting better

UE: So angry

UN: So frustrated

Chin: No one understands

CB: So scared I'll never get better

UA: When I saw progress I worked more

TOH: I loved seeing progress

EB: When I saw progress I had hope

SOE: When I have hope I keep going

UE: I like having hope

UN: I wonder if I can have hope again?

Chin: I am open to feeling hope

CB: I love the feeling of hope

UA: Hope makes me feel stronger

TOH: Hope gives me energy

EB: I love the feeling of energy

SOE: When I have energy I keep going

UE: I am open to the possibility I still can make progress

UN: I like how I feel when I'm making progress

Chin: I want to believe I can make progress

CB: But I don't want to be a fool

UA: Other people make progress

TOH: I could make progress

EB: I could be a miracle story

SOE: I don't know if I could be a miracle

UE: Maybe I'm afraid of being a miracle

UN: Maybe I'm afraid I'll be disappointed

Chin: I'll just be disappointed now and save myself the trouble

CB: Maybe I am a miracle

UA: Maybe I'm not a miracle

TOH: If I am or am not a miracle, *I still am me*

EB: I am me and I am alive

SOE: If I'm alive, I am growing

UE: If I am growing, I am making progress

UN: If I am making progress I am getting better

Chin: I like getting better

CB: I like growing

UA: I wonder what new thing will enable me to grow more?

TOH: I'm open to seeing, hearing and learning what new thing I could do or could be to move me to the next stage?

Take a deep breath, and feel the energy shift. This is a resourceful state.

Once you are in this renewed and resourceful state, you can begin to think of different goals and different ways to achieve them. For example: Change your exercise routine: if you were using weights, try bands, find new energizing music, choose a new location, get a workout partner, search for a new therapist, get feedback from a support group. Be willing and open to defining a new goal.

Get resourceful first.

ESSENTIAL TAKEAWAYS

- *Apparent* plateaus become real only when you think there is no more progress and you disengage.
- Disengagement leads to decline.
- Question what else might be causing a "stuck state."
- Get in a resourceful state before you plan new goals.
- Apparent plateaus are a call to *change it up* not give up.
- Consider tapping, meditation, journaling, speaking with a counselor, social worker, online survivor group, or taking a nap to get in a more resourceful state.

FORGIVENESS, ACCEPTANCE, & REINVENTION (C&S)

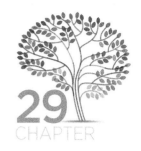

> *To forgive is to set a prisoner free*
> *and discover*
> *that the prisoner was you.*
> **~ Lewis B. Smedes ~**

FORGIVENESS

The concept of forgiveness previously existed only in the realm of spirituality and religion, not in medicine or science. But scientists studying the mind-body connection have begun asking, "How do our emotions affect our DNA, the very blueprint for who we are and the instructions for who we will become?"

The evidence is clear. Harboring anger, resentment, and hate are physiologically bad for your body because these emotions activate our stress response. Dawson Church, Ph.D., founder of the National Institute for Integrative Health and the author of *The Genie in Your Genes,* cites numerous scientific researchers, neuroscientists, and medical doctors who explain what happens to our genes in response to psycho-emotional changes. He states, "The circulation of these stress hormones through your system on a regular basis will compromise your immune system, weaken your organs and age you prematurely."

An overly stressed nervous system produces excess cortisol, adrenaline, and glucose as a means of preparing the body to fight or flee. Since we are not usually utilizing those hormones to actually fight or flee, they circulate in the body. When excess glucose circulates, it leads to insulin resistance, which can lead to Type 2 Diabetes in the long run. When diabetes is uncontrolled, it can lead to a devastating cascade of serious health issues including kidney failure, vision issues, and an increased risk of heart attack and stroke. Simply stated, negative emotions put the body in a chronic state of stress, the result of which may increase your risk for stroke because these emotional states also elevate blood pressure and increase inflammation in the arteries.

What triggers chronic stress? Trauma, loss, mistreatment, abuse, injustice, betrayal, fear, financial problems, caregiving, self-imposed and other people's expectations. Traumas large and small often have their origins in childhood. Even a child living in a stressful environment is unknowingly modifying their DNA.

Nearly everyone has experienced some version of a violation from simple name-calling to egregious and unspeakable acts of harm. The greater the violation, the more logical it seems to justify hatred and resentment. Why would anyone *want* to forgive a perpetrator?

It may not be readily apparent why forgiveness isn't actually about the perpetrator, but in reality it's a healing tool for you, the one who has been harmed. Forgiveness is *not*, however, about ignoring the harm done to you or about giving consent to allow harm to persist. *The process of forgiveness is intended to relieve you of the repetitive and recurrent insult that keeps your trauma and bitterness alive and in present time.*

WHEN YOU ARGUE WITH THE PAST, YOU KEEP IT ACTIVE

Ironically, we inadvertently keep our own trauma, abuse, or injustice alive and current by reliving events and having conversations about it. You will know how active and current it is by the way you feel. Our *attention* to these awful, unjust acts magnifies their presence and harms us.

I've heard stroke survivors speak angrily about doctors who seemed uncaring and dismissive, and one who couldn't forgive the doctor who nicked an artery resulting in his stroke. There have been others who felt hurt, betrayed, and abandoned by a spouse, friend, or employer who no longer wanted a relationship with them. These situations are painful and real. There's no doubt they've happened, so why or how could forgiveness be considered?

Remember the oft-quipped statement: "*Harboring hate and anger is like drinking poison while expecting the other person to die.*"

HOW FORGIVENESS HEALS

Why consider forgiveness? Because it is a tool for freeing yourself and allowing your body to heal. Even mainstream medicine now recognizes the benefits of forgiveness.

According to psychiatrist Dr. Karen Swartz, director of the Mood Disorders Adult Consultation Clinic at John Hopkins Hospital, "There is an enormous physical burden to being hurt and disappointed." Studies have shown that forgiveness can greatly benefit your health, lowering the risk of heart attack, improving cholesterol levels and sleep, and reducing pain, blood pressure, and levels of anxiety, depression, and stress.

The Mayo Clinic says this: "Letting go of grudges and bitterness can make way for improved health and peace of mind. Forgiveness can lead to: healthier relationships; improved mental health; less anxiety, stress, and hostility; lowered blood pressure; fewer symptoms of depression; a stronger immune system; improved heart health; and improved self-esteem."

If those promised health benefits are appealing to you, then forgiveness is at least worthy of curiosity. If we break apart the word FOR-GIVE, we may look at forgiveness with new eyes. Ask yourself: are you *for-giving*? Are you *for-giving* yourself improved mental health and wellbeing? Are you *for-giving* yourself lower blood pressure? Are you *for-giving* yourself peace of mind?

Dr. David Levy, a highly respected endovascular neurosurgeon who performs some of the most complicated and dangerous brain surgeries, shared this insight in his book, *Gray Matter*: "When I first began praying for patients, I had no idea that it would lead me to discover the power of forgiveness. The idea that bitterness was the source of health problems would not have made sense to me earlier in my career, but over time I became convinced that one of the greatest thieves of joy and health is the unwillingness to forgive the people who have hurt you."

Dr. Levy shares numerous stories of his patients who said that when they allowed themselves to forgive, they felt "freed," and their most common remark was, "I feel tremendous peace."

While forgiveness may mean different things to different people, it is generally a personal and conscious decision to *let go of resentment and thoughts of revenge.* It may be a process you can achieve with the guidance of clergy or a psychologist, but it can also be achieved through journaling, prayer, tapping, and other techniques. See Appendix Resources under Mental Health/ Surrendering Technique.

Only you have your finger on your DNA switch. Are you *forgiving* yourself a chance to flip that switch and gain peace of mind and healing?

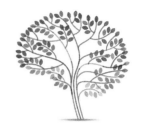

ACCEPTANCE

Find a place inside where there's joy,
and the joy will burn out the pain.
~ Joseph Campbell ~

Acceptance, as you recall, according to Elisabeth Kübler-Ross, is the last stage of grief and loss. It's also perhaps the most challenging. The belief that "What you resist not only persists, but will grow in size" is a common tenet of psychology. When we resist *what is*, we suffer. But why and how does one *accept* unwanted circumstances?

Acceptance can feel like passively giving up or succumbing to something undesired with the belief that your circumstance will be unchanging. But what if instead of acceptance we said *acknowledgement*? *Acknowledging* where you are at any given moment in time is important.

Think of getting a flat tire in the middle of a rainstorm, at night, by yourself on the freeway. You can resist it, bargain, scream, curse, and blame, but until you acknowledge you have a flat and take the steps to change your circumstance to the best of your ability, you will suffer. Yes, I realize a tire is not your life, but you can only ever be where you are. That doesn't mean you will always be there. In fact, it's impossible to *not* change. We are all changing every moment of every day, and our thoughts and feelings contribute greatly to the direction of this change.

What is, is already old news. "It" already happened. Acknowledgment and acceptance are the vehicles that make room for transformation and allow for the conscious choice of exploring the most pressing question... "What's next?"

I can't tell you how, when, or *if* you will achieve acceptance. I can only tell you that those who have achieved it open new chapters in their lives. I know this *can* happen. It has happened for millions of people. It is the turning point for moving beyond loss and grief and towards what is possible. *I believe this can happen for you.*

My words are of little value. I am only a guide. This, after all, is *your journey.* I will leave the bottom of this chapter full of white space. This is the space for you. When the time is right, you will write the chapter of your acceptance.

What Acceptance Means to Me

REINVENTION

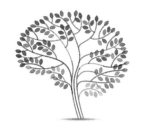

*We must be willing to let go of the life we planned
so as to have the life that is waiting for us.*
~ Joseph Campbell ~

Nobody chooses having a stroke as a plan to reinvent their career path, their marriage, or their outlook on life. In the game of life, a stroke is like a giant reshuffling of cards. Reinvention is only possible when one chooses to stay in the game and play that new hand, regardless of the cards dealt.

Reinvention is on the other side of acceptance.

Remember Jean, whose first words after her stroke were "NOT YET!"? She yelled this in response to her doctor's suggestion that her family should sell her condo because he thought she'd never be able to care for herself.

How did Jean deal with her newly shuffled cards? Her journey of ups and downs, growths and insights, spanned eight years. Her "thousand-mile journey" began, as Lao Tzu said, with "a single step" and was achieved exactly one day at a time.

At first, Jean worked on healing her body while dealing with the grief and loss that accompanied her awareness of her new self. She transitioned from a caregiver to a care receiver. This transition was hardest on her self-esteem and challenged her deepest fear and belief that she would be *not* be cared for except through her own efforts. Allowing and accepting care when she was helpless gave her an "incredible inner peace and trust that the universe provides."

As Jean shed her old life, she dealt with the hit it took on her identity as a professional; it was tough giving up the psychotherapy practice she'd worked hard to build.

However, when she let go of that, she saw something new—a need for stroke survivors that wasn't being filled. Jean helped establish the Rocky Mountain Stroke Association in Colorado. In addition, she founded the Stroke Visitation Program with peer counseling, a program that's helped hundreds of survivors as well as The Nurturing Place: A Stroke Assistance Center. At age 78, 40 years after her stroke, Jean says her energy level seldom limits her. She still even privately counsels one stroke survivor.

Jean realizes each person's definition of a "quality life" is very subjective. She says, "I'm delighted to notice that the term 'stroke' no longer has much meaning to me, either as an illness I have or as a definition of myself. Yes, I'm still hemiplegic and walk using a cane and an ankle-foot orthotic. Yes, I still have a slight aphasia when I think faster than I can express my thoughts. And yes, I sometimes have word-finding difficulties (which my friends remind me, could be age; but that's another topic). But these just seem like characteristics of myself now, no more or less important than being five feet tall, having auburn hair, and light skin."

Most importantly, Jean says, "I am back to not just enjoying my life, but savoring it. I feel I am just where I should be. Through the creation of the Rocky Mountain Stroke Association, the Stroke Visitation Program, and The Nurturing Place, I've come full circle; from needing total care to now being able to guide others as they, too, rise to the challenge of developing changed but quality lives."

Connor was an accomplished architect and designer. He was educated, well-traveled, an exceptional cook, and an expert gardener who grew his own fruits, vegetables, and herbs. Connor and his wife had a large circle of foodie friends who got together for evenings where Connor held court as the erudite, sharp-witted storyteller. His stroke left him paralyzed on the right side of his body and severely aphasic. Connor was easily agitated, very frustrated, and angry. He'd explode with anger perseverating on a single word when he wasn't understood. His anger often led to shortened sessions as Connor huffed out of the room red-faced and shaking his head.

Connor eventually learned to walk more independently using a walker and then a cane. He learned to say a few phrases, answer questions more spontaneously, and even use an iPad tablet with limited success for communication. What Connor found, though, was art.

Connor returned to painting, but this time it was with his nondominant hand. His artwork became a tremendous source of pleasure and self-esteem. He felt whole and worthy engaging in an activity in which he was completely independent. He found meaning, purpose, and joy in this medium. He was commissioned to paint canvases for a woman who staged houses for real estate showings, enabling him to feel both significance and contribution. He continued having dinner with friends and travelling to the family's Palm Springs home, and when he felt overloaded or fatigued, he'd excuse himself and retire to a quiet place. Connor's wife learned to become more independent, too, allowing Connor time to himself when he didn't want to attend concerts in the park, an activity they both previously loved.

Valerie Greene was a healthy 31-year-old on the fast track to becoming a millionaire. She had a thriving business as an estate planner where she served her clients with the utmost integrity. She drove a nice car, lived at a posh address, had a personal trainer, and was in top physical condition. By many standards, *she had it all*.

While at her office one day Valerie had a crushing, sudden, and severe headache isolated on one side of her head. She thought she just needed to relax, so she left the office for home thinking a warm shower might help. In the shower, things got worse. A wave of dizziness and nausea swept over her, causing her to sink to the floor. She barely managed to open the shower door, reach for her phone, and dial 911. Firemen rushed her to the hospital, and after undergoing an MRI, the results concluded Valerie suffered a *migraine*.

Valerie followed up with the physician who'd seen her at the hospital. Her MRI showed an *irregularity*, but because of her age and apparent good health, the irregularity was dismissed as a false positive reading. Valerie sought the advice of a neurosurgeon who happened to also be a client. He suggested repeating the MRI, and while Valerie respected his opinion, she was in no hurry to repeat that "claustrophobic and time-consuming procedure."

Over the course of the next six months, Valerie had two more emergency room visits and three misdiagnoses. She didn't have a migraine. She didn't have vertigo, and she didn't have multiple sclerosis. She had actually suffered a minor stroke, but she still didn't know that, nor did anyone else.

Ten days later, on June 10, 1996, a very large blood clot formed; it totally blocked her *basilar artery*, the superhighway where all routes to the brain merge into one. By all medical terms, Valerie should not have lived.

Valerie had a massive brain stem stroke that paralyzed the left side of her body. She lost most of her hearing and was unable to speak. Doctors told her that she might never walk or talk again.

Barely able to blink, she lay lifeless on a hospital bed, paralyzed, drooling, and scared. At that point, according to her, she thought, "I knew my fate was in the hands of my creator."

Valerie's doctors misdiagnosed more than her condition. They also misdiagnosed her character and her inner strength. They didn't know that her faith, deeply instilled within her as a child, grounded her resolve and determination.

As for getting her life back? Valerie purposefully decided she didn't want to get her old life back. Instead, she embraced and welcomed the new life that awaited her. Admittedly, it was painful and sobering at times, watching her colleagues and friends excel in their lives because, in contrast, she was shedding everything of "value," including selling her house, her furniture and all of her belongings in order to receive the best care possible. Valerie knew her life was spared for a reason and that something amazing was in her future. And was it ever.

It's said that what doesn't kill you makes you stronger, and Valerie's experience is proof.

Having survived 2 strokes at age 31 that paralyzed her and robbed her of the ability to speak, she held fast to the belief that her life had a purpose and plan. Determined to heal, she spent years regaining her abilities, one piece at a time.

Today, Valerie is a worldwide symbol of hope, a two-time published author, a national speaker, and the founder of a world outreach (Global Stroke Resource, Inc., also known as Bcenter.org). Valerie is known as "America's Stroke Coach," and she has a private practice offering personal coaching to survivors and families.

After nearly three decades, her life's work and purpose continue to share hope and healing with her fellow stroke survivors around the world. Her vision is to build a world-class stroke recovery center that will become the top global destination for stroke recovery. The Florida headquarters is currently in its planning stages with completion anticipated for fall 2023.

This is how Valerie put it: "Yes, my life was forever changed the day I suffered a stroke. But instead of choosing to let it rob my future, it became a gift to let others know they are not alone and to never give up! Remember, we are not in control. So let go and let God."

Dr. Jill Bolte Taylor is perhaps the best-known stroke survivor in the world today. At the age of 37, this Harvard-trained brain scientist had a massive left-hemisphere stroke. When she first realized she was having a stroke, she recalled thinking, "How cool is this? How often does a brain scientist get to study her brain from the inside out?" Her story of reinvention goes beyond her physical recovery and delves deeply into finding her way to a different level of consciousness and the "circuitry of deep inner peace."

In both her book, *A Stroke of Insight*, as well as her *must-see* TED Talk, (already viewed over eight million times), Dr. Taylor describes with exquisite clarity how her left brain hemisphere progressively shut down, causing her to lose all functional abilities related to walking, talking, speaking, writing, and memory. However, it was that very dysfunction that allowed her access to her right hemisphere where she felt "a sense of euphoria, wellbeing, and peace" she'd never experienced before.

Dr. Taylor's story has universal appeal perhaps because, in her own words, it is about "the beauty and resiliency of our human brain and its innate ability to constantly adapt to change and recover function."

Dr. Taylor's complete recovery took eight years, but she shares her progressive milestones, noting the things that most helped her recover, including the importance of people focusing on what she *could do* versus her disabilities, celebrating any and all small successes every day, and defining her priorities for what she wanted.

Like many stroke survivors, Dr. Taylor ultimately viewed her stroke as a "blessing," a comment heard by many survivors who find meaning and insight as an unexpected side effect of their trauma. Dr. Taylor wrote, "This stroke of insight has given me the priceless gift of knowing that deep inner peace is just a thought/feeling away."

There are as many stories of reinvention as there are survivors. Whether one volunteers at a place of interest, returns to work, creates a new opportunity providing a solution for survivors' unmet needs, or is simply a member of a family or support group, the *story* of reinvention doesn't matter as much as *the person matters.*

***The you that you are* is what matters.**
You are here for a purpose.

PARTING WORDS

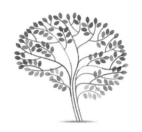

We've come to the end of this book, but surely not the end of *your* story. I am awed by the privilege, honor, and trust given to me as your partner and guide during this time. Most importantly, though, I hope that through the course of our connection, you have gained the knowledge, confidence, and belief in yourself that you're capable and equipped to manage this journey. I pray that you continue to keep hope as your pilot light and that you find and make a life worth living.

You began this journey scared, confused, and in need of answers. You were an explorer in unknown territory, but as promised, you've become an expert. No expert knows all the answers—it is their *questions* that make them experts. You've learned to ask powerful questions. There is more to your journey. Get ready to fly.

We'll end as we began...

Take a breath. Close your eyes and tell yourself aloud...

"Yes, I can."

"Yes, I must."

"Yes, I will."

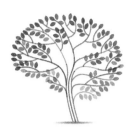

APPENDIX
RESOURCES THAT MAKE LIFE EASIER

ORGANIZATIONS

The sites below have valuable information and links to stroke prevention, stroke education, associated services, clinical trial studies, and ways for caregivers and survivors recovering from stroke to be supported and involved.

American Heart Association (AHA)
www.heart.org
(800) 242-8721

American Speech-Language-Hearing Association (ASHA)
www.asha.org
(800) 638-8255
Provides directory of speech/language pathologists and audiologists.

American Stroke Association (ASA)
www.StrokeAssociation.org
(888) 478-7653
Provides free magazine, *Stroke Connection,* for caregivers and survivors.

American Stroke Foundation
www.americanstroke.org
The American Stroke Foundation's Stroke Survivor Navigation Program offers intensive support to help survivors and their

caregivers adjust to life after stroke. Stroke survivors who are within six months of their stroke are eligible for this free program. Through weekly telephone calls, survivors and caregivers can address adjustment issues encountered at home, examine ways to avoid a second stroke, and learn about new community resources. If you think you might be interested in this program, call the Stroke Survivor Navigation Program at (913) 213-5493.

National Aphasia Association

www.aphasia.org

(800) 922-4622

Provides constantly updated and delineated information for caregivers and survivors about aphasia and stroke in an easy-to-navigate website.

National Easter Seal Society

www.easterseals.com

(800) 221-6827

Provides information and services to help people with disabilities. Offers caregivers respite care. Provides day programs for adults and children.

National Institutes of Health (NIH)

www.nih.gov

The National Institutes of Health is a part of the U.S. Department of Health and Human Services. NIH is the largest biomedical research agency in the world. Their researchers make important discoveries that improve health and save lives. Their site provides information regarding mental and physical health conditions and medications searchable by name. It also presents new research and lists clinical trials.

National Stroke Association (NSA)

www.stroke.org

Stroke Helpline: (800) 787-6537 (1-800-STROKES)

Provides free magazine, *Stroke Smart,* for caregivers and survivors. Provides information on prevention and treatment for caregivers and survivors. Provides directory of Stroke Center locations throughout the U.S. Offers online support including how to start a support group, group registry, e-publications, webinars, iHOPE, and Living After Stroke.

Rehab Without Walls® (RWW)

www.rehabwithoutwalls.com/services/stroke-rehabilitation/

Rehab Without Walls® home and community rehab blends evidence-based therapies with creative uses of the patient's own surroundings – whether at home, school, work or in their own community. Home and community neuro therapy programs are covered by some commercial health insurance and workers' compensation plans. Medicare does not cover home and community-based rehabilitation. Contact for locations where services are available.

Stroke Clubs International

(409) 762-1022

Maintains a list of over 800 stroke clubs throughout the United States. Call for the name and contact information of a stroke club in your area.

CLINICAL TRIALS AND STUDIES

Research studies often recruit survivors for participation in tests of new drugs and therapies. You may find a research program for participation based on your location or by type of study and eligibility qualifications. For information and questions about clinical studies, visit the following reputed websites.

Barrow Neurological Institute

www.barrowneuro.org/patients-families/

(800) 227-7691

A regional specialty center in Phoenix, Arizona, Barrow Neurological Institute is one of the premier destinations in the world for neurology and neurosurgery. Their website provides links to clinical trials.

Department of Health and Human Services

https://ClinicalTrials.gov

For more information about what a clinical trial is and how it operates, visit their Frequently Asked Questions (FAQs) page here: *https://clinicaltrials.gov/ct2/about-studies/learn.*

National Institute of Neurological Disorders and Stroke (NINDS)

www.ninds.nih.gov/Disorders/Clinical-Trials/Find-Ninds-Clinical-Trials?province=CA&field_disorders_taxonomy_tags_tid=Stroke &page=2

Worldwide Studies

https://clinicaltrials.gov/search/term=Stroke

CAREGIVER RESOURCES

Caregiver Action Network

www.caregiveraction.org

The nation's leading family caregiver organization. Provides information on caregiving, video products, and many other caregiver resources.

The Evidence-Based Review of Stroke Rehabilitation (EBRSR)

www.ebrsr.com

A website for research, The Stroke Rehabilitation Evidence-Based Review (SREBR) reviews techniques, therapies, devices, procedures, and medications associated with stroke rehabilitation. More geared to researchers than lay people.

The Well Spouse Association

https://wellspouse.org

(800) 838-0879

Provides support for the husbands, wives, and partners of people who are chronically ill or disabled.

FOOD WEBSITES THAT HELP ORGANIZE MEAL SUPPORT AND OTHER FORMS OF ASSISTANCE

Care Calendar

www.carecalendar.org

- Allows you to schedule services beyond meals, like housework, running errands, and childcare. Gives maps and driving directions to recipient(s).

Lotsa Helping Hands

http://lotsahelpinghands.com

- Very simple and user-friendly
- Helps you coordinate care, meals, and support
- Provides simple templates to request services

Can create a community in 60 seconds.

Meal Train

www.mealtrain.com

- Offers a "How it Works" demo and sample meal plan
- Provides a message board for communicating with the recipient and other contributors
- Sends email reminder to participants before their scheduled day
- Meal Train *Plus*: For a one-time $10 fee (for the duration of use), services such as childcare, housework, lawncare, and rides can also be scheduled.

Take Them a Meal

https://takethemameal.com

- Offers sample schedule
- A Bowl of Good program allows participants to order meals and have them delivered (frozen) to the recipient. Available in 24 of the 50 United States, primarily in the northeast, Midwest, mid-Atlantic, and southeastern parts of the country.

You may already have some people helping in one or more of these categories, but if not, you can use the services listed above or any of the links to templates to send a personalized email letter to those who've offered and whom you trust.

CAREGIVER TEMPLATES

Template: Email Ask for Help

http://bit.ly/2RA0Kii

Template: Menu of Activities

http://bit.ly/2s9Q2AC

DRIVING RESOURCES

The Association for Driver Rehabilitation Specialists (ADED)

www.aded.net/default.aspx

(866) 672-9466

Established in 1977 to support professionals working in the field of driver education/driver training and transportation equipment modifications for persons with disabilities through education and information dissemination.

State-by-State Requirements for VIP (Handicap) Placard

www.verywellhealth.com/handicapped-parking-permit-189676

Sure Grip

http://suregrip-hvl.com/about.html

Founded by Keith Howell, who became quadriplegic in his early teens and later developed a set of controls to emulate the easiest style of driving. Sure Grip hand controls have become a leader in the disabled driving aids market in both Canada and the U.S.

DYSPHAGIA/EATING AIDS

Frazier Free Water Protocol

www.fvfiles.com/521200.pdf

Instructions on how to use the water protocol for survivors who are restricted from drinking water. Use this sheet to consult your speech pathologist and physician *before* trying this protocol on your own. **May not be suitable for all survivors due to aspiration risk.**

National Foundation of Swallowing Disorders

https://swallowingdisorderfoundation.com

Offers in-person local support groups across the country. They offer two online support groups; one for adults with dysphagia and one for parents/caregivers of infants and children with feeding & swallowing disorders. They also provide resources including videos, brochures, peer-to-peer mentoring, and swallow exercises.

Puree Food Molds

www.pureefoodmolds.com/en/6-silicone-puree-food-molds

Food molds that provide real food shapes for puree diet.

FINANCIAL ISSUES

Patient Advocate Foundation

www.patientadvocate.org

(800) 532-5274

Helps patients dealing with chronic, life-threatening, or debilitating diseases. Services include mediation to assure access to quality health care, maintaining employment, and preserving financial stability to help ease the burden of medical debt. All services are free.

Prepare to Care

www.aarp.org/caregiving/prepare-to-care-planning-guide.html

An online tool developed by AARP that manages the challenges of survivor finances affected by issues related to medical insurance, as well as the potential cost of accessibility-improving home renovations and long-term care.

Smart About Money (SAM)

www.smartaboutmoney.org

A program of the National Endowment for Financial Education (NEFE), a nonprofit national foundation dedicated to inspiring empowered financial decision-making for individuals and families through ups and downs at every stage of life.

MEDICAL INSTITUTIONS

U.S. News & World Health Report's:
10 Best U.S. Rehabilitation Hospitals

- **Shirley Ryan AbilityLab
  (formerly Rehabilitation Institute of Chicago)**
  Chicago, IL 60611-2654
- **Spaulding Rehabilitation Hospital, Massachusetts
  General Hospital**
  Charlestown, MA 02129-3109
- **TIRR Memorial Hermann**
  Houston, TX 77030-3405
- **Kessler Institute for Rehabilitation**
  West Orange, NJ 07052-1424
- **Mayo Clinic**
  Rochester, MN 55902-1906
  (507) 405-0312
- **Rusk Rehabilitation at NYU Langone Hospitals**
  New York, NY 10016-6402
- **Craig Hospital**
  Englewood, CO 80113-2899
- **Shepherd Center**
  Atlanta, GA 30309-1465
- **MossRehab**
  Elkins Park, PA 19027-2220
- **New York-Presbyterian Hospital-Columbia and Cornell**
  New York, NY 10065-4870

MEDITATION, MINDFULNESS, TAPPING, AND TOOLS FOR INNER PEACE

EFT Universe: Dawson Church

www.eftuniverse.com

Tapping information. Many free resources, including videos and tap-along sequences. Free EFT manual download. Resource directory for locating practitioners in your area.

Emotional Freedom Technique: Original Creator Gary Craig

www.emofree.com

Many free resources including a download of the EFT manual as well as Personal Peace Procedure Tapping point chart and videos. Resource directory for locating practitioners in your area.

Downloadable Chart for Meridian Points for Tapping

https://bit.ly/2GWIiw8

Strategies for Reducing Sensory Overload in Social Settings: A Blog Post

https://blog.constanttherapy.com/18-tips-for-survivors-strategies-for-reducing-sensory-overload-in-social-settings

The Tapping Solution App

(Available for Apple)

The app is free to download and offers a *limited selection of free tapping topics* including anxiety. It provides visual and verbal instructions with a way to rate and track your progress. *Fees apply to access the full library that changes every six months.*

The UnLonely Project

www.artandhealing.org

Promotes social connection through the arts. See their website for their interactive Film Fest and UnLonely music playlist and changing events.

MINDFULNESS APPS FOR IPHONE & ANDROID

Search for these on your phone

Calm

Free trial. The selections range from 3-minute to 25-minute sessions. Breathing exercises and sleep stories.

Headspace

Free trial. Good for beginners. Uses a buddy system, and applies meditation to life.

Insight Timer

Free. More than 4,500 free guided meditations from over 1,000 practitioners.

The Mindfulness App

Free trial. Five-day guided meditation practice. Many sounds to choose from and can have guided or silent meditations with ambient sound.

Sattva Meditations and Mantras

Free. Motivates you to meditate every day. Preloaded exercises including timers and chants. Plus, you can check your heart rate via the app and participate in challenges.

NUTRITIONAL SUPPORT

American Diabetes Association

www.diabetes.org
(800) 342-2383
Website offers extensive information about food, fitness, and lifestyle management for diabetes.

American Dietetic Association (ADA)

www.eatright.org
(800) 877-1600
Consumers may speak to a registered dietitian for answers to nutrition questions or obtain a referral to a local registered dietitian. Website offers sample calorie-controlled menus.

Ilyse Wasserman Petter, MS, Founder of *LettuceB*

Clinical nutritionist specializing in vegan diets.

https://lettuceb.organic

Lindsey Layton, Holistic Health Coach

www.purefit.live

www.lindseylayton.com

(502) 396-6349

Certified American Association of Drugless Practitioners (AADP) coach specializing in bio-individuality diet programs. Offers complimentary 20-minute phone consultation.

OCCUPATIONAL THERAPY AIDS

Help for Arm and Hand

Adaptive Clothing

www.silverts.com

Clothing for those with limited arm mobility.

Flint Rehab

www.flintrehab.com

Products from this company are built with neuroplasticity in mind, knowing that repetition builds networks. For instance, MusicGlove ($349) is a hand rehabilitation device clinically proven to improve hand function in two weeks. It works by motivating users to perform hundreds of therapeutic hand and finger exercises while playing an engaging musical game. Log onto their website to request a free consultation to determine if the product is appropriate.

Flint Rehab also offers FitMi ($299), home computer-assisted physical therapy exercises for the whole body. (Does not work with iPad.) FitMi contains two wireless pucks and a therapy app that picks exercises for you tailored to your stage of recovery. As you improve, the FitMi exercises and difficulty levels increase to optimize your recovery.

One Hand Can

www.onehandcan.com

A stroke survivor who's created kitchen tools for one-handed cooking. She has video demonstrations on her website.

One-Handed Tools and Tricks: An Article

www.strokenetwork.org/newsletter/products/tools.htm

"Day to Day Survival" is a useful article by David Wasielewski, a hemiplegic stroke survivor and columnist for Stroke.net. His article helps the hemiplegic survivor learn tricks to choose easy garments for dressing, manage closets, showers, baths, and bathroom dispensers, stairs, walkways, and more.

Stroke Rehab: A Guide for Patients & Their Caregivers

www.stroke-rehab.com

Stroke Rehab is a downloadable eBook (no hard copy available) written by an OT with over 20 years of treatment experience. The book retails at $14.95 and includes techniques of stroke rehabilitation to use at home, over 130 photos, easy exercises, and suggestions for adaptive and home exercise equipment.

PHONES FOR SURVIVORS

California Telephone Access Program (CTAP Free Adaptive Phones)

www.californiaphones.org

Offering free specialized phones to Californians who are deaf, hard of hearing, speech disabled, blind, or who have low vision, cognitive impairments, or restricted mobility. These persons are eligible to receive equipment with certification by a medical doctor, a licensed audiologist or speech-language pathologist, a qualified state agency, or a hearing aid dispenser. *Check with your state to determine if they have a similar program.*

PHYSICAL THERAPY/CONSTRAINT INDUCED THERAPY (CIT)

The Anat Baniel Method

www.anatbanielmethod.com

Constraint-Induced Therapy (CIT)

> ***Please note: participation in CIT or mCIT requires a survivor to have some limb mobility.***

Multiple clinics are listed

- **The Taub Therapy Clinic** Behavioral neuroscientist Edward Taub, Ph.D., and his research group at the University of Alabama at Birmingham (UAB) originated Constraint-Induced Movement Therapy (CI therapy, or CIMT), with the first human study published in 1993. Over the past 25 years, Dr. Taub and his research and clinic staff have further developed and refined CI therapy. *taubclinic@uabmc.edu*
  https://www.uabmedicine.org/
  (866) 554-8282

- **CI Therapy Research Group** Please contact Staci McKay in the UAB CI Therapy Research Group at (205) 934-9768 to learn about the studies that are underway now. University of Alabama at Birmingham
  1720 2nd Ave South,
  CPM 712,
  Birmingham, AL 35294
  Phone: (205) 934-9768
  citherapy@uab.edu

- **Modified CIT (mCIT)** A less intense treatment that involves the same principles as CIT (i.e., restraint of the less-affected upper extremity and practice of functional activities with the more-affected extremity), but with less intensity and shorter sessions than traditional CIT. The common therapeutic factor in all CIT techniques includes concentrated, repetitive tasks with the more-affected arm.

- **Kessler Institute for Rehabilitation, West Orange, NJ**
  www.kessler-rehab.com
  (973) 731-3600
- **Advanced Recovery Rehab Center**
  www.advancedrecovery.org
- **Mary Free Bed**
  https://www.maryfreebed.com/patients-visitors/contact-us/
  235 Wealthy St. SE
  Grand Rapids, MI 49503
  (616) 840.8000
  (800)528.8989

The Feldenkrais Method

https://feldenkrais-method.org

SEX RESOURCES

American Association of Sexuality Educators, Counselors and Therapists (AASECT)

www.aasect.org

Dallas Novelty

www.dallasnovelty.com/about-us/

Purveyor of sex toys for people of different abilities. Ships within the U.S.

Kait Scalisi, MPH, Sex Educator

www.passionbykait.com

Many resources for sex toys, mindful sex, orgasm resources, and personal consultation.

Dr. Mitchell Tepper, Certified Sexuality Educator and Counselor, Author of *Regain That Feeling*

www.drmitchelltepper.com

SLEEP

Dr. Michal J. Breus, The Sleep Doctor

The personal sleep doctor for Dr. Oz. His website offers informative blogs, quizzes, and resources for improving sleep.

https://www.thesleepdoctor.com/

SPEECH THERAPY PROGRAMS, APPS, AIDS, SUPPORT GROUPS

A downloadable e-book about aphasia available through Lingraphica

https://devices.aphasia.com/thank-you-aphasia-journey-ebook?submissionGuid=858e2e90-ef26-426c-80bd-1a4a972873b8

Aphasia Friendly

www.aphasiafriendly.co

Many free downloadable pictures and speech therapy resources, including printable wallet cards for people with aphasia.

Constant Therapy

http://constanttherapy.com

iPad platform-based therapy with a growing library of 58 science-based task categories and over 12,000 exercises. For home practice with or without a speech therapist. **Prices:** 30-day free trial. Individual Patient/Caregiver: $19.99 monthly; $199.99 yearly; $349.99 for three years.

Holistic Speech-Language Pathologists

Bright Side Therapy, LLC

www.brightsidetherapy.com
jen@brightsidetherapy.com

Bright Side Therapy offers language and cognitive treatment materials, a dysphagia recipe cookbook, aromatherapy, mindfulness education and brain health coaching services to maximize your recovery.

Tsgoyna Tanzman, MA/CCC-SLP
Master Practitioner of NLP, Certified Life Coach
www.hope-stroke.com/
hopeafterstrokenow@gmail.com

Tsgoyna has helped thousands of people transition after stroke and brain injury to the next stages of their lives. With more than 25 years of experience, she is an expert at helping people find both the inner and outer resources needed for the process of recovery combining traditional speech therapy with life coach practices and techniques from Neurolinguistic Programming. Tsgoyna specializes in working with clients on functional and integrative strategies for finding meaning and purpose in their lives. Can provide teletherapy and coaching via Zoom or Facetime.

Lingraphica

www.aphasia.com

Many resources including a printable wallet card for identifying aphasia. Lingraphica offers three dedicated communication devices for adults with aphasia. All three devices are backed by research and reimbursable by Medicare and many private insurances. The laptop model, the *AllTalk*, is also available with *EyeGaze* technology to help individuals with physical limitations who need a hands-free device to communicate. The two tablet models, the *TouchTalk* and the *MiniTalk*, are designed for a mobile and active lifestyle while providing an easy way to communicate. All devices come with a specialized new source, 17 voices, email and instant messaging capabilities, and therapy activities to help strengthen speech and language skills. **Price:** *Free trial,* reimbursable by Medicare.

Lingraphica SmallTalk Apps

www.aphasia.com/products/communication-and-practice-apps

An augmentative family of free apps for practicing speech and communicating on the go. Common graphic icons, phrases, and videos help adults with aphasia communicate whatever they need. The site is free to use from the web or the TalkPath Therapy app. Clinicians can also link accounts with their clients and manage their plans of care straight from the app or computer. **Platforms:** iPod touch, iPhone, iPad. **Price:** Free.

Lingraphica E-book about aphasia

https://devices.aphasia.com/thank-you-aphasia-journey-ebook?submissionGuid=858e2e90-ef26-426c-80bd-1a4a972873b8

Minnesota Connect Aphasia Now (MnCAN)

http://www.mncan.org/

http://www.facebook.com/MNConnectAphasiaNow

612-524-8802

MnCAN is a non-profit dedicated to helping people with aphasia improve their quality of life to live fully within their communities. Programs include conversation groups for persons with aphasia and educational programs for those with primary progressive aphasia. Care partner support groups are also available. Each MnCAN conversation group is facilitated by a Speech-Language Pathologist (SLP) and volunteers or SLP grad students who use conversation strategies to support effective communication. Fall and Winter sessions meet for 12 weeks, Summer sessions meet for 8 weeks. See website for specific sites and more information.

Proloquo2Go

www.assistiveware.com/product/proloquo2go

Proloquo2Go is an Augmentative and Alternative Communication (AAC) application for iPad, iPhone, and iPod touch that provides a "voice" for people who have difficulty speaking or cannot speak at all. It's suitable for children, teenagers, and adults who need symbol support to communicate. Most likely a person will need training to optimize function for full and robust communication. **Platforms:** iPad, iPhone, and iPod. **Price:** $219.99.

Support Groups on Facebook

You can join any and all of these groups after introducing yourself and agreeing to the conditions of the group. These groups offer peer to peer support and discussions of problems and solutions. Survivors often share leading edge knowledge of equipment and programs that have aided in their recovery. You can find these groups by searching these names on Facebook.

- **I am Proud to be a Stroke Survivor**
- **Life After Stroke**
- **Stroke Recovery at Home**
- **Young Stroke Survivors Global Network**

TactusTherapy

www.tactustherapy.com

Offers a wide range of speech therapy apps for adults with aphasia and other communication challenges. These evidence-based apps are designed by a speech-language pathologist to be used in the clinic and at home. Easy to use and affordable to own. Tactus Therapy apps have no subscriptions, login screens, or need for Wi-Fi. Use the App Finder to find the best apps for your needs. **Platforms:** iOS and Android mobile devices. **Price:** Varies per app ($5-$25) with discount bundles available. Free lite versions to try.

Tapgram

www.tapgram.com

Tapgram makes sending simple messages to your loved ones easy. Once you are set up, you won't need to touch a keyboard to send messages to the people that you love. Instead, you create messages by tapping on images, and the messages can be posted to your social media feed or sent to your friends and loved ones via email. In turn, friends and family can tap on pictures to send you a reply. You will need a phone, tablet, or a computer with a connection, and a free Tapgram account. It comes with a quick start guide. **Platforms:** phone, tablet, computer. **Price:** Free.

Teletherapy TalkPathLive

https://www.talkpathlive.com/what-we-do/

855-274-9582

Provides affordable, state-of-the-art online speech-language therapy to individuals of all ages, with all types of communication challenges, including: language, articulation, fluency, voice/resonance, and swallowing. Every program is supervised and evaluated by a certified SLP for clinical effectiveness. Call to discuss therapeutic options.

SOOTHING GAMES AND DISTRACTIONS

Free Apps available on Apple or Android

- Flower Cells
- Candy Crush

TRAVEL/BATHROOM NEEDS

"Travel John"

www.traveljohn.com

Disposable urinals. Sanitary, personal urinals containing "LiQsorb®." Turns liquid urine into an odorless gel for ease of disposal. Unisex adapter makes it easy for female use as well. Must use while sitting (providing there is the use of gravity with an unobstructed, free-flowing opening) or standing, with a spill guard to prevents backflow during use.)

Where to Use: On car trips. On planes (yes, you can discreetly pee under a blanket in your seat). Anywhere an accessible bathroom is unavailable.

Why I Like It: Easy to use, turns a messy problem into NO problem. It's cheap and *not* a handicapped aid, but a truck driver's lifesaver. Travel John is only for liquid waste, *not for solid.*

Cost: $4.95.

GLOSSARY OF TYPES OF STROKES

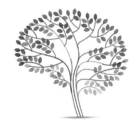

Reprinted with Permission: Moawad, H. (2017, July) 'Types of Strokes." *verywell health*. Retrieved from: *https://www. verywellhealth.com/types-of-stroke-3146303*

There are many different types and categories of stroke. Types of stroke are described by two main criteria- their location and by the cause of tissue damage in the brain.

Cause of Tissue Damage

Strokes can be caused by a variety of factors. Often the causes can help determine the prognosis as well as the best method of treatment. A stroke may result from a blood clot interrupting blood flow in the brain, by a bleeding blood vessel in the brain, or by low blood flow to a region of the brain.

Blood Clot-Ischemia

A stroke caused by a blood clot is called an ischemic stroke due to the lack of blood supply, and thus oxygen and vital nutrients, to a region of brain tissue. An ischemic stroke may be caused by an embolus, which is a blood clot traveling from another part of the body. It may be caused by a thrombus, usually as a result of cerebrovascular disease. Or, it may be the result of vasospasm, the sudden severe narrowing of a blood vessel in the brain.

Hemorrhagic

Bleeding of a blood vessel in the brain causes a hemorrhagic stroke. Sometimes the rupture of a brain aneurysm causes bleeding. Extreme changes in blood pressure may trigger the rupture of a brain aneurysm. Sometimes a region of the brain that has been damaged by ischemia can bleed within the first few days after a stroke, causing a secondary hemorrhage.

Watershed Stroke

A watershed stroke is caused by low blood pressure or low blood flow that compromises blood supply to susceptible areas of the brain. A watershed stroke may occur in regions of the brain that are supplied by tiny arteries.

Location

Strokes are also described by their location because the affected part of the brain corresponds to specific neurological or behavioral deficits.

Cortical Stroke

A cortical stroke affects the cerebral cortex, which controls high level processing. Different parts of the cerebral cortex control different functions.

Frontal Cortex

A frontal lobe stroke often causes muscle weakness on the opposite side of the body and trouble with decision-making. People with a stroke involving the frontal cortex may display socially inappropriate behavior, paranoia or may regress in maturity. Occasionally, loss of bladder or bowel control may result.

Parietal Cortex

The parietal cortex is involved with integration of sensation and language. People with a parietal stroke often display impaired sensation or trouble with the production of speech.

Occipital Cortex

The occipital cortex integrates vision. A stroke in this region may cause complete or partial loss of vision on the opposite side of the occipital region affected.

Temporal Cortex

The temporal cortex is involved with hearing and language. People who have had a temporal lobe stroke often have trouble understanding written or spoken language.

Subcortical

A subcortical stroke affects the deeper regions of the brain.

Thalamic

A thalamic stroke usually causes significant sensory deficits on the opposite side of one or more parts of body, even when the stroke affects a relatively small region of the brain.

Internal Capsule

A stroke affecting the internal capsule may affect motor or sensory function of one or more parts of the opposite side of the body.

Brainstem

A brainstem stroke can cause a wide variety of signs and symptoms. It may cause weakness, sensory changes, or trouble speaking. A brainstem stroke can affect the movement of the opposite side or the same side of the face or mouth. People who experience a brainstem stroke may have trouble with eye movements, which often manifests as double vision or blurred vision. Additionally, the brainstem controls breathing and regulates the heart rate. A brainstem stroke may affect vital functions, even when a relatively small area is affected.

Blood Vessel

Some strokes are named after the blood vessel that was blocked or bleeding. The most commonly identified blood vessel in a stroke is the middle cerebral artery, which often causes a large cortical stroke affecting the temporal and parietal lobes.

GLOSSARY OF TERMS

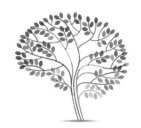

Abulia: Abulia shows up as a lack of concern about one's condition or the world around a person. In extreme cases, a person with abulia may become mute even though they may be able to speak. Abulia is clinically distinct from depression. People with abulia typically do not exhibit signs of sadness or negative thoughts. Your doctor must help differentiate the disorders as the treatments are very different.

Active Assisted Range of Motion (AAROM): Therapists use active assisted range of motion exercises (AAROM) to help the survivor who has some ability to move but still needs help to practice the exercises or complete the movement. A therapist may help guide the movement with their own body (hold the limb, for example) or use bands and other exercise equipment.

Acute Phase of Recovery: The first seven days after the onset of symptoms of a stroke. The brain is in a delicate stage. Keep the survivor calm and safe. Limit stimulation and visitors. Follow passive range of motion (PROM) exercises. Look for spontaneous recovery (improvement with no effort), as it signals the start of the subacute phase.

Ambulatory: Able to walk, even if using an assistive device, such as a cane or walker.

Amygdala: A tiny, almond-shaped network of neurons that is a component of the limbic system, the amygdala triggers our fight-or-flight response, also known as the stress response. The limbic system is located in the midbrain, between the frontal lobes and the hindbrain (also called the reptilian brain—the most primitive part of the brain.) The limbic system is the source of emotions and long-term memory.

Aneurysm: An aneurysm occurs when an artery wall weakens and causes an abnormally large bulge. This bulge can rupture and cause internal bleeding. Although an aneurysm can occur in any part of the body, they're most common in the brain.

Aphasia: Aphasia is an impairment of language, affecting the production or comprehension of speech and the ability to read and/or write. Aphasia is always due to injury to the brain, most commonly from a stroke, particularly in older individuals. See Chapter 7 for a full description of the varying types and severity ratings of aphasia.

Apraxia: Apraxia is a condition in which the mouth's muscles are strong, but a person has lost the ability to *volitionally sequence* motor movements. Apraxia may occur orally (a person may stick out his tongue when asked to blow a kiss), verbally (a person may not be able to repeat words because he cannot volitionally match the sequence of sounds to make words), or it can occur in limbs (a person may comb his hair in response to being asked to gesture brushing his teeth.) Limb apraxias make it hard for a person with apraxia (PWA) to use gestures to supplement their missing speech simply because they can't get their limbs to do what they want even if they are able to conceptualize an intended gesture.

Aspiration Pneumonia: Aspiration pneumonia is a lung infection that occurs when food, saliva, liquids, or vomit are breathed into the lungs or into the airways leading to the lungs instead of being swallowed into the esophagus and stomach. This infection can lead to fatal consequences if not treated.

AVM: Arteriovenous malformation (AVM) is a *congenital disorder* (present at birth) of blood vessels in the brain, brain stem, or spinal cord that is characterized by a complex, tangled web of abnormal arteries and veins connected by one or more *fistulas* (abnormal communications). Aneurysms and AVMs are often called the brain's ticking time bombs, because these abnormalities of the vessels may be present at birth, but have no symptoms until they suddenly burst.

Bio-individuality: Bio-individuality, a term coined by the Institute for Integrative Nutrition, suggests that no two people are alike and that each of us has unique food and lifestyle needs, so no single food philosophy or diet can yield the same results for everyone.

Bolus: A small, rounded mass of a substance, especially of chewed food at the moment of swallowing. May also refer to a single dose of a drug or other medicinal preparation given all at once especially in tube feedings.

Bone Flap: A surgical procedure in which a flap is created in a flat bone by leaving one side of a rectangle cut in the bone intact. The procedure is used for gaining access to a cavity, often the brain. Specialized tools are used to remove the section of bone called the bone flap. The bone flap is temporarily removed, then replaced after the brain surgery has been done. The bone flap may reside in a patient's abdomen until swelling subsides and can be replaced on the skull.

Chronic Phase of Recovery: On the stroke timeline, the chronic phase of recovery begins three months after stroke and continues for the rest of your life.

Coherence: The state of being highly ordered, organized, and efficient. In a coherent system all individual parts operate in harmony.

Cognition: Conscious process of knowing or being aware of thoughts or perceptions including understanding and reasoning.

Cognitive Impairment: Difficulty with perception, memory, attention, planning, reasoning skills, judgement, impulse control, self-regulation, flexibility, goal persistence, self-awareness, task initiation, time management, and/or organization. Cognitive impairment affects one's ability to engage in activities of daily living such as hygiene, eating, household management, community re-integration, driving, and so on.

Commode: A bedside commode is a movable toilet that does not use running water. It looks like a chair with a toilet seat and has a bucket or container underneath. The container can be removed for cleaning after the commode is used. A commode can be placed beside the bed if a person cannot get to the bathroom.

Contracture: A condition resulting from chronic spasticity wherein a joint is flexed for too long and the soft tissue hardens. A contracture is a shortening and hardening of muscles, tendons, or other tissue, often leading to deformity and rigidity of joints.

Contralateral: Means on the *opposite side*. Brain damage in the left hemisphere affects body parts on the right side or contralateral side.

Brain damage in the right hemisphere affects body parts on the left side or contralateral side.

Craniectomy: A craniectomy procedure includes the removal of a bone flap, but in this case, it is not returned to its location after the procedure is finished. This may be due to trauma to the bone itself because the brain is too swollen to permit the return of the bone flap or because the surgeon feels it is in the patient's best interest. If there is an infection in the area, for example, the bone flap may be discarded.

Craniotomy: A craniotomy is a surgery during which a piece of the skull called a bone flap is removed in order to allow a surgeon access to the brain.

CT Scan: A computerized tomography (CT) scan combines a series of X-ray images taken from different angles around the body and uses computer processing to create cross-sectional images (or slices) of the bones, blood vessels, and soft tissues inside the body. CT scan images provide more detailed information than plain X-rays do.

Decision Fatigue: Refers to the deteriorating quality of decisions made by an individual after a long session of decision-making. It often results in making poorer decisions that default to comfort.

Disinhibition: The loss of inhibition. This may show up as saying inappropriate things or exhibiting inappropriate behaviors especially of a sexual nature.

Dysarthria: Speech that is characteristically slurred, slow, and difficult to understand as a result of motor impairment. The oral muscles are weak or paralyzed and can't form words. Think about what it feels like to have a massive Novocain injection at the dentist—decreased or absent sensation and weak or paralyzed muscles in the mouth. The tongue has eight muscles. The lips and cheeks also have muscles that help with speech production, chewing and moving food into a ball (*bolus*) in preparation for swallowing. When these muscles are weak or paralyzed, a person may slur words, drool, dribble food from their mouth, trap food in the pockets of the cheek, and have swallowing problems because they can't form food into a ball and push it toward the back of the mouth.

Dysphagia: A swallowing disorder that may occur because of weak or paralyzed muscles or because of a breakdown in the sequencing and timing of the complex swallow reflex.

HOPE AFTER STROKE *For Caregivers and Survivors*

Edema: Swelling. A condition characterized by an excess of watery fluid collecting in the cavities or tissues of the body.

EFT: Emotional Freedom Technique (EFT), also known as "Tapping" is an evidence-based therapeutic tool recognized by the American Psychological Association that helps lessen anxiety, stop the stress response, and reduce the stress hormone, cortisol. It makes use of a technique that combines Cognitive Behavioral Therapy (exposure and talk therapies) with acupuncture meridians (tapping on the energy meridians that run through our bodies without the use of needles.). Tapping, is the physical act of using percussive tapping movements on various acupuncture meridian endpoints to deactivate the stress response (sympathetic nervous system) and activate the relaxation response (parasympathetic nervous system) for the purpose of reducing anxiety, fears, and pain. Tapping is a quick and painless self-help approach that can be used anywhere at any time. Trained practitioners are best at leading a person in a session, but an individual can learn to use tapping as a self-help tool. For more information, use this link:*www.eftuniverse.com.*

Esophagus: The part of the alimentary canal that connects the throat to the stomach.

Flaccid: Weak or limp. Paralysis in which muscle tone is lacking in the affected muscles and in which tendon reflexes are decreased or absent.

Hemiparesis: Partial paralysis of half of the body including the head, arm, leg, and trunk on either the left or right side.

Hemiplegia: Total paralysis of half of the body including the head, arm, leg, and trunk on either the left or right side.

Hemorrhage: Bleeding or the abnormal flow of blood.

Hippocampus: The hippocampus is a part of the limbic system. The limbic system is the area in the brain that is associated with memory, emotions, and motivation. The limbic system is located just above the brainstem and below the cortex. The hippocampus itself is highly involved with our memories.

Holistic: Treatment of the whole person, taking into account mental and social factors rather than just the physical symptoms of a disease.

Humerus: The bone of the upper arm or forelimb, forming joints at the shoulder and the elbow. The shoulder blade (*scapula*) and the upper arm bone (humerus) come together to form the shoulder joint. This joint is shaped like a ball and socket. When a paralyzed arm hangs, the weight of it can cause the joint to partially dislocate or separate. This is called a *subluxation*.

Hyperacute Phase of Recovery: On the stroke timeline, it is the first six hours after the onset of a stroke.

Hypoxia: A lower-than-normal concentration of oxygen in arterial blood, as opposed to *anoxia*, a complete lack of blood oxygen. Hypoxia will occur with any interruption of normal respiration.

Inflammation: The body's natural response to protect itself against harm. There are two types of inflammation: acute and chronic. Acute inflammation protects the body from invaders such as viruses, bacteria, and microbes. Chronic inflammation damages cells. Chronic inflammation can occur in response to other unwanted substances in the body, such as toxins from cigarette smoke or an excess of fat cells (especially fat in the belly area). Chronic inflammation causes *atherosclerosis*—the buildup of fatty, cholesterol-rich plaque that eventually narrows arteries and limits blood flow. If the plaque breaks off the artery wall and mingles with blood, it may form a clot that blocks blood flow. These clots are responsible for the majority of heart attacks and most strokes.

Intracerebral hemorrhage (ICH): ICH is caused by bleeding within the brain tissue itself—a life-threatening type of stroke. ICH is most commonly caused by hypertension, arteriovenous malformations (AVM), or head trauma.

Intracranial Pressure: A measurement of the pressure of brain tissue and the cerebrospinal fluid that cushions and surrounds the brain and spinal cord. An increase in intracranial pressure can be due to a rise in pressure within the brain, which may in turn be caused by bleeding into the brain, fluid around the brain, or swelling within the brain itself.

Learned Nonuse: This is the result of trying and failing a movement so often (e.g., trying to open and close a hand) that the stroke survivor believes their effort is futile, and the part of the brain that controls that movement shrinks.

Lacunar Stroke: Lacunar stroke is a type of ischemic stroke that occurs when blood flow to one of the small arteries deep within the brain becomes blocked. According to the National Institutes of Health (NIH) lacunar strokes represent about one-fifth of all strokes.

Limbic System: The limbic system is located in the midbrain, between the frontal lobes and the hindbrain (also called the reptilian brain—the most primitive part of the brain.) The limbic system is the source of emotions and long-term memory.

Mirror Neuron: Mirror neurons are a type of brain cell that responds equally when we perform an action and when we witness someone else perform the same action. An example of this is yawning when someone else yawns.

Mirror Therapy: Mirror therapy is used to stimulate an affected limb to mimic the movements of a healthy limb by means of triggering mirror neurons to fire. When one sees the illusion of his affected arm moving in the mirror, even though it's just a reflection of the functioning arm, studies have shown that the brain perceives it as the affected arm and mobility can improve. See this video for a demonstration: *www.youtube.com/watch?v=GNanQtMBwys*

MRI: An MRI (magnetic resonance imaging) lets your doctor see the organs, bones, and tissues inside your body without having to do surgery. This test can help diagnose a disease or injury. You might need an MRI if an X-ray or CT scan didn't give enough information about your condition. An MRI of the brain helps your doctor diagnose an aneurysm and stroke. A special kind of MRI called a functional MRI (fMRI) checks brain activity by measuring blood flow to certain areas of your brain.

Neologism: Jargon or made-up words commonly seen with Wernicke's aphasia.

Neuro-fatigue: Severe mental fatigue not necessarily relieved by rest. Scientists have confirmed through PET scans that stroke survivors recruit more brain areas in performing normal activities than they did before their brain injury. This means they require more energy to do what they previously did. Parts of the brain that previously showed little activity while performing a specific action now become actively involved through many extra bypass areas. In other words, it takes more brain energy to accomplish the same task.

Neuroplasticity: Neuroplasticity is the brain's spectacular capacity to change and reorganize itself by growing new neural pathways and synaptic connections. "Neuro" means neuron. "Plastic" stands for changeable, malleable, modifiable.

NG Tube: Nasogastric tube. A feeding tube that goes down the nose to the stomach. Feeding tubes are given to people who are either comatose, barely alert, and/or have demonstrated swallowing problems that cannot be resolved quickly or do not allow for the patient to receive adequate nutrition by mouth safely. Nasogastric tubes are inserted for short- or medium-term nutritional support not to exceed six weeks.

Orthotic: An orthopedic appliance or apparatus used to support, align, prevent, or correct deformities or to improve the function of movable parts of the body. Also known as braces, splints.

PBA: Pseudobulbar affect (PBA) is a secondary neurologic condition of stroke that causes excessive, sudden, unpredictable, inappropriate or uncontrollable laughing or crying that doesn't match how one feels. Other emotional outbursts like agitation, impulsivity, and disinhibition may also be the result of frontal lobe damage and are not considered within the normal, expected range of emotions. It is different than depression and must be diagnosed by a doctor to receive proper treatment.

Penumbra: The area surrounding the core, or the spot where nerve cells (*neurons*) die as a result of a stroke. The penumbra is the area of recovery because its cells are thought to be stunned, not dead. In the early stages of recovery the penumbra begins to resolve.

PEG Tube: PEG (percutaneous endoscopic gastrostomy) tubes require a minor surgical procedure wherein a feeding tube is inserted directly into the stomach. PEG tubes are inserted when long-term dysphagia renders oral eating unsafe. Although PEG tubes reduce the chance of aspiration pneumonia, people can still aspirate on non-oral feedings. It's critical to make sure your LO remains in an upright position for any tube feeding to lessen the risk of reflux, regurgitation, and aspiration. PEG tubes also require specific care to maintain hygiene and lower the risk of infection at the skin site.

Physiatrist: A special rehab medicine doctor who is versed in the latest stroke recovery treatments. The physiatrist is the gatekeeper of the rehab team and is responsible for ordering tests and directing therapeutic services including all therapists or other specialists throughout the rehab process.

Plateau: A word used to describe a flattening out of progress in which a survivor appears to have stopped making recovery progress. It can relate to progress in either or all of the following areas: speech, occupational, or physical therapy. Apparent plateaus may be overcome by a change in treatment modalities or shifts in medications or other factors that otherwise improve mental persistence.

Premorbid: Refers to what happened before the stroke.

PROM (Passive Range of Motion): Passive means without active participation of a survivor. A physical therapist may perform passive range of motion (PROM) exercises to maintain a paralyzed limb's muscle length and joint flexibility without the active participation of the survivor. Often this is done immediately post-stroke and before active therapy can begin.

Proprioception: Proprioception means "sense of self," knowing where the body is in space. A sense or perception, usually at a subconscious level, of the movements and position of the body and especially its limbs, independent of vision. In the limbs, the proprioceptors are sensors that provide information about joint angle, muscle length, and muscle tension, which are integrated to give information about the position of the limb in space. The sense of proprioception is critical to safe walking.

PWA: An acronym for Person With Aphasia. Rather than referring to a person as an aphasic, it reminds us aphasia is a condition a person *has,* not who they *are.*

Scapula: Also known as the shoulder bone, shoulder blade, wing bone, or blade bone, the scapula is the bone that connects the *humerus* (upper arm bone) with the clavicle (collar bone).

Spasticity: A condition in which certain muscles are continuously contracted. This contraction causes stiffness or tightness of the muscles and can interfere with normal movement, speech, and gait. Spasticity is usually caused by damage to the portion of the brain or spinal cord that controls voluntary movement. Temporary measures to help reduce spasticity include both oral and injectable medications. Permanent improvement, however, relies on re-establishing brain control over spastic muscles.

Subacute Phase of Recovery: On the Stroke Timeline, the subacute phase is the period from seven days to approximately three months from onset of stroke. It is the most important phase for stroke recovery because neurons are coming alive. Stimulation, therapy, and neuroplasticity lead to the highest level of recovery. This is known as the "Use It or Lose It" period.

Subarachnoid Hemorrhage: A subarachnoid hemorrhage (SAH) is a bleed into the space between the brain and the skull. The subarachnoid space is a potential space. It normally contains cerebrospinal fluid. An SAH occurs as a result of an artery on or near the surface of brain bursting. A SAH may be genetic and present at birth or can occur as a result of a fall or other head trauma.

Synergies: This refers to abnormal patterns of motor movement wherein one uses *bundled* movements of multiple joints, to accomplish something usually done by one joint. For example, a person uses their elbow, shoulder, and hand as a unit to accomplish the *simple* act of bending just their hand.

Tapping: Tapping, also known as EFT, Emotional Freedom Technique, is an energy-based treatment modality accepted by the American Psychological Association. It is the physical act of using percussive tapping movements on various acupuncture meridian endpoints to deactivate the stress response (sympathetic nervous system) and activate the relaxation response (parasympathetic nervous system) for the purpose of reducing anxiety, fears, and pain. Tapping is a quick and painless self-help approach that can be used anywhere at any time. Trained practitioners are best at leading a person in a session, but an individual can learn to use tapping as a self-help tool. See *www.eftuniverse.com*.

Tone Management: Tone refers to our muscular tension and responsiveness to a stimulus. An increase of tone is often caused by spasticity, the abnormal muscle stiffness due to damage in the brain and/or spinal cord. Tone management can be achieved through physical therapy, the Feldenkrais Method® and the Anat Baniel Method®.

TpA: Tissue plasminogen activator (TpA) is a powerful clot-busting drug. It works by dissolving the clot and improving blood flow to the part of the brain being deprived of blood. Alteplase IV r-tPA needs to be used within 3 hours of having a stroke or up to 4.5 hours in certain eligible patients. The earlier tPA is administered within that time frame, the better the chances of a favorable outcome are. If given promptly, one in three patients who receive tPA resolve their symptoms or have major improvement in their stroke symptoms.

Trachea: Often referred to as the windpipe, it is a cartilaginous tube that connects the pharynx and larynx to the lungs, allowing for the passage of air. In swallowing problems, food, liquid, or bacteria in saliva can enter the trachea and go into the lungs, causing aspiration. If the particles can't be expelled with a normal cough reflex, it can lead to aspiration pneumonia.

Videofluoroscopic Swallowing Study (VFSS): VFSS, also known as modified barium swallow, is a radiographic procedure that provides a direct, dynamic view of oral, pharyngeal, and upper esophageal function during swallowing. The test can diagnose where and what the problems are during the act of swallowing. Proper diagnosis is necessary to determine the most appropriate treatment measures to prevent aspiration pneumonia. The barium is necessary to view structures via videofluoroscopy during the swallow.

Visual Field Cut: *(Information obtained from the Stroke Association.)* "Strokes often affect vision and processing of visual information. The most common visual deficit is *hemianopia* or visual field cut. Our visual field is the whole area that we see in front of us — left to right, top to bottom. Each eye has its own visual field, but the brain combines the information from both eyes so we only see the world as one visual field. Like so many processes in the brain, vision in one eye is processed on the opposite side of the brain, but it isn't as simple as the left eye being handled by the right brain. Instead, visual stimulation from the left side of each eye is handled in the right visual cortex. Right-side stimulation of each eye is processed in the left visual cortex. The visual cortex is located in the back part of the brain (refer to the link to see *How Vision Works*). A stroke that injures either the optic nerves running from the back of the eyeballs through the brain to the visual cortex or the visual cortex itself will cause a deficit of vision in the same area of both eyes. Thus, a stroke in the visual processing area of the right side of the brain causes a problem with the left visual field of the right eye and the left visual field of the left eye. For an easy-to-understand infographic, refer to this link to understand visual field cuts. Often specialized glasses with prisms may help in eliminating visual field cuts. Contact a *neuro-optometrist* for treatment in optometric training and proper evaluation for glasses: *http://strokeconnection.strokeassociation.org/Winter-2017/From-the-Eyes-of-the-Beholder/.*"

Visual Neglect: Visual neglect or hemispatial neglect is a neuropsychological condition in which, after damage to one hemisphere of the brain, a person exhibits a deficit in attention to and awareness of one side of their field of vision. Common observable characteristics of this problem include not seeing things on one side that may cause a survivor to bump into things on the affected side. The survivor will not see objects or people on the affected side of vision. Often food is completely ignored on the side of the plate where vision is affected. This is a serious concern for driving and must be corrected before a survivor can safely drive.

INDEX

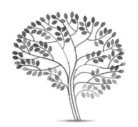

A

abulia *111, 305*
active assisted range of motion
    exercises (AAROM *99*
active range of motion exercises
    (AROM) *94*
activity of daily living (ADL)
    stroke recovery *32, 212*
acute phase
    stroke recovery *14–17, 24*
ambulatory condition
    physical therapy *112*
amygdala
    anatomy *165–167*
Anat Baniel Method
    physical therapy *95–96*
aneurysm *1, 10, 41, 208–209*
anxiety *4, 104, 116–118, 120, 162,*
    165–166, 171–173, 183, 194, 269
aphasia
    speech therapy *35, 41, 51, 52, 56,*
        69–71, 74, 77, 150, 171, 209,
        214, 236
apps (smartphone)
    resources and tools *41, 74–75,*
        82, 111, 161
apraxia
    speech therapy *35, 78–80, 82,*
        209

arteriovenous
    type of stroke *10*
aspiration pneumonia
    feeding and swallowing disorders
        86

B

bio-individuality
    nutrition *191*
blockage
    type of stroke *17–19, 141*
bolus
    feeding and swallowing disorders
        77, 87
bone flap *50, 53*
brain bleed
    type of stroke *11, 17*

C

Chronic Phase
    stroke recovery *15, 261*
clinical depression (see also:
    depression) *143, 181*
commode *137*
constraint-induced therapy (CIT)
    occupational therapy *34*
contracture
    physical therapy *101*

D

decision fatigue *178*
dietary changes
 nutrition *190–191*
dietitian
 nutrition *190–191*
disinhibition
 personality changes *116–117*
driving
 stroke recovery *43, 52, 54, 77,*
  104–106, 112, 149, 171, 218,
  227, 233
Driving
 stroke recovery *245*
dysarthria
 speech therapy *35, 77, 209*
dysphagia
 feeding and swallowing disorders
  35–36, 85

E

edema *11, 197*
Emotional Freedom Technique
 Tapping *167, 173, 289*

F

feeding tubes
 feeding and swallowing disorders
  90–92
Feldenkrais Method
 physical therapy *95–96*
Frazier Water Protocol (or "Free
 Water Protocol")
 feeding and swallowing disorders
  90

G

gratitude
 mindfulness *4, 47, 49–50, 144,*
  154–156, 159, 177, 178, 183,
  228
Gratitude
 mindfulness *192*

H

health insurance
 case management *21, 32, 36, 40,*
  55, 105, 136, 169, 247
hemiparesis *87*
hemiplegia *87*
hemorrhagic stroke
 type of stroke *10, 157*
high blood pressure *10, 60, 207*
hippocampus
 anatomy *167*
Hippocampus
 anatomy *309*
Hyperacute Phase
 stroke recovery *15*

I

intracerebral hemorrhage
 type of stroke *111*
ischemic stroke
 type of stroke *12, 43–44, 141*

J

Jill Bolte Taylor
 Thrivers *95, 277*

L

learned nonuse *40, 45*
limbic system
 anatomy *165–166*

M

meditation
 mindfulness *140–141, 144, 160,*
  195
Meditation
 mindfulness *178*
mirror neurons *78, 223*
mirror therapy *101*

N

neuroplasticity
 stroke recovery *15–17, 93–95,*
  95, 176, 180, 217–219

Norman Doidge, M.D.
    stroke experts *16, 95*
nutrient-dense food *189*
nutritionist *190, 194*

O

occupational therapist *32–33, 39, 86,*
    137, 172, 212
omega-3 fatty acids
    nutrition *186, 189, 193*
orthotic device
    physical therapy *35, 274*

P

passive range of motion (PROM)
    exercises *18, 94, 99*
PEG tubes
    feeding and swallowing disorders
    91
penumbra
    stroke recovery *12–16, 30*
physiatrist *32, 40, 44*
physical therapist *32–34, 94–95, 179*
proprioception *94, 198*
pseudobulbar affect (PBA) *117, 182*

R

recurrent stroke *60, 140–141*

S

sexual intercourse
    love and intimacy *4, 205–211*
smoking *119, 140, 179, 207, 237–238*
spasticity
    physical therapy *97–102, 212,*
    245, 250
speech therapist *1, 14, 32, 33, 56, 74,*
    79, 80, 86
spontaneous recovery
    stroke recovery *15, 18, 30, 45,*
    261

Standard American Diet
    nutrition *186, 190*
subacute phase
    stroke recovery *15, 121, 217*
subarachnoid hemorrhage
    type of stroke *11*

T

tantra yoga
    love and intimacy *214*
tapping (see also: Emotional
    Freedom Technique)
    anxiety treatment *4, 104, 116,*
    120, 162, 165–167, 171, 173,
    183, 194
Thrivers *47–48, 53–54, 240*
tone management
    physical therapy *34*
tPA *13, 43, 141*
transient ischemic attack (TIA)
    type of stroke *11, 42–43*

V

Valerie Greene
    Thrivers *xiii, 231, 275*
visual neglect *149*
vitamins for stroke recovery and
    prevention
    nutrition *193–194, 196*

Y

yoga
    mindfulness *144, 179*

BIBLIOGRAPHY

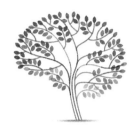

1. "About Dr. Mitchell Tepper." *Dr. Mitchell Tepper.* 2016. Web. *www. drmitchelltepper.com/about.*

2. Adan, A. "Cognitive performance and dehydration." *Journal of the American College of Nutrition.* 31.2 (2012): 71-8. Print.

3. "Aphasia Statistics." *National Aphasia Association.* 2016. Web. *www. aphasia.org/aphasia- resources/aphasia-statistics/.*

4. Baniel, Anat. "Dr. Jill Bolte Taylor Taking Anat Baniel Method NeuroMovement Training." *Vimeo.* 15 Sept. 2017. Web. *https://vimeo. com/234075110.*

5. Bolte Taylor, Jill. *My Stroke of Insight: A Brain Scientist's Personal Journey.* New York: Penguin Books, 2006. Print.

6. Brady, Adam. "The Coherent Heart: 3 Steps to Accessing Heart Intelligence." *The Chopra Center.* Web. *https://chopra.com/articles/ the-coherent-heart-3-steps-to-accessing-heart- intelligence.*

7. Breus, Michael. "The Newest Science on the Sleep and Health Benefits of CBD." *The Sleep Doctor.* 6 November 2018. *www.thesleepdoctor.com/2018/11/06/ the-newest-science-on-the-sleep-and-health-benefits-of-cbd/.*

8. "Caregiving in the U.S. 2009." National Alliance for Caregiving, AARP. Nov. 2009. Web. *www.caregiving.org/data/Caregiving_in_the_ US_2009_full_report.pdf.*

9. Castillo, Brooke. "Ep. #204: Cognitive Dissonance." *The Life Coach School.* 22 Feb. 2018. Podcast. *https://thelifecoachschool.com/204/.*

10. *If I'm So Smart, Why Can't I Lose Weight?* Scotts Valley, CA: Book Surge LLC [CreateSpace], 2006. Print.

11. Chan, Amanda. "Sex, coffee increases risk of brain aneurysm rupture." *NBC News*. 9 May 2011. Web. *www.nbcnews.com/id/42963765/ns/ health-health_care/t/sex-coffee-increases-risk- brain-aneurysm-rupture/*.

12. Church, Dawson. *The Genie in Your Genes: Epigenetic Medicine and the New Biology of Invention,* 2nd edition. Santa Rosa, CA: Energy Psychology Press, 2009. Print.

13. Clarey, Christopher. "Olympians Use Imagery as Mental Training." *New York Times*. 22 Feb. 2014. Web. *www.nytimes.com/2014/02/23/sports/ olympics/olympians-use-imagery-as- mental-training.html*.

14. Clear, James. *Atomic Habits: Tiny Changes, Remarkable Results*. New York: Penguin Books, 2018. Print.

15. Cuddy, Amy. "Your Body Language May Shape Who You Are." *TED Conferences LLC*. June 2012. Web. *www.ted.com/talks/ amy_cuddy_your_body_language_shapes_who_you_are*.

16. Davis, G. Albyn. "Aphasia Therapy Guide." *National Aphasia Association*. Feb. 2011. Web. *www.aphasia.org/aphasia-resources/ aphasia-therapy-guide/*.

17. Davis, Jeanie Lerche. "Meditation Balances the Body's Systems." *WebMD*. 1 Mar. 2006. Web. *www.webmd.com/balance/features/ transcendental-meditation#1*.

18. "Depression." *National Stroke Association*. 2018. Web. *www.stroke.org/ we-can-help/survivors/ stroke-recovery/post-stroke-conditions/emotional/ depression*.

19. Doidge, Norman. *The Brain That Changes Itself: Stories of Personal Triumph from the Frontiers of Brain Science*. New York: Penguin Books, 2007. Print.

20. *The Brain's Way of Healing: Remarkable Discoveries and Recoveries from the Frontiers of Neuroplasticity*. New York: Penguin Books, 2015. Print.

21. Dong, Hongli, et al. "Efficacy of Supplementation with B Vitamins for Stroke Prevention: A Network Meta-Analysis of Randomized Controlled Trials." *PloS One* 10.9 (2015): e0137533. doi:10.1371/journal. pone.013753.

22. Drillinger, Meagan. "Meet the Paralyzed Man Making Sex Toys for People with Disabilities." *Men's Health*. 12 Jan. 2018. Web. *www.menshealth.com/sex-women/a19546493/ sex-toys-for- people-with-disabilities/*.

23. Ellis, Ian Justl. "The Structure and Function of the Epiglottis." *SLR EM Education*. Vimeo. 25 Feb. 2015. Web. *https://binged.it/2x0TfVa*.

24. Elrod, Hal. *The Miracle Morning: The Not-So-Obvious Secret Guaranteed to Transform Your Life Before 8AM.* Hal Elrod, 2012. Print.

25. "Fatigue." *National Stroke Association.* 2018. Web. *www.stroke.org/we-can-help/survivors/ stroke-recovery/post-stroke-conditions/physical/fatigue.*

26. Fogarty, Lisa. "8 Ways to Bang Out an Orgasm With a Partner without Actually Having Penetrative Sex." *She Knows.* 23 Jun. 2017. Web. *www.sheknows.com/love-and-sex/articles/1058865/8-ways-to-get-off-without-sex/.*

27. "Foods that fight inflammation." *Harvard Health Publishing.* Harvard University. Published June 2014. Updated 7 Nov. 2018. Web. *www.health.harvard.edu/staying-healthy/ foods-that-fight-inflammation.*

28. Fordyce, Moira. "Caregiver Health." *Family Caregiver Alliance.* Web. *www.caregiver.org/ caregiver-health.*

29. "Forgiveness: Letting Go of Grudges and Bitterness." *Mayo Clinic.* 4 Nov. 2017. Web. *www.mayoclinic.org/healthy-lifestyle/adult-health/in-depth/forgiveness/art-20047692.*

30. "Forgiveness: Your Health Depends on It." *Johns Hopkins Medicine.* Web. *www.hopkinsmedicine.org/health/healthy_aging/healthy_connections/forgiveness-your-health-depends-on-it.*

31. Frankl, Viktor. *Man's Search for Meaning.* Boston: Beacon Press, 2006. Print.

32. Fuchs, Eberhard, and Gabriele Flügge. "Adult Neuroplasticity: More than 40 Years of Research." *Neural Plasticity.* (2014). Web. *http://dx.doi.org/10.1155/2014/541870.*

33. Grossman, Stan. "Nearly Half of Acute Stroke Patients are Dehydrated." *Neurology Advisor.* International Stroke Conference 2015 coverage. 12 Feb. 2015. Web. *www.neurologyadvisor.com/ isc-2015-coverage/acute-stroke-dehydration/article/397842/.*

34. "iHOPE: Sex and Sexuality after a Stroke." *National Stroke Association.* 13 May 2013. Web. *www.stroke.org/stroke-resources/resource-library/ihope-sex-and-sexuality-after-stroke.*

35. "Impact of Stroke (Stroke Statistics)." *American Stroke Association.* Web. *www.strokeassociation.org/STROKEORG/AboutStroke/Impact-of-Stroke-Stroke-statistics_UCM_310728_Article.jsp#.XAqnLhNKh8U.*

36. James, Matt. "Conscious of the Unconscious." *Psychology Today.* 30 Jul. 2013. Web. *www.psychologytoday.com/us/blog/focus-forgiveness/201307/conscious-the-unconscious.*

37. Kwah LK, and RD Herbert. "Prediction of Walking and Arm Recovery after Stroke: A Critical Review." *Brain Sciences.* 6.4 (2016): 53. Print. doi:10.3390/brainsci6040053.

38. Lamola G., F. Bertolucci, B. Rossi, and C. Chisari. "Clinical Assessments for Predicting Functional Recovery after Stroke." *International Journal of Neurorehabilitation.* (2015). 2:174.doi:10.4172/2376-0281.1000174.

39. Lava, Neil. "Brain Swelling." *WebMD.* 16 Sept. 2018. Web. *www.webmd. com/brain/brain- swelling-brain-edema-intracranial-pressure#1.*

40. Layton, Lindsey. Personal Interview. 10 November 2018

41. Leape, Lucian. "Error in Medicine." *JAMA* 272.23 (1994): 1851-1857. Print.

42. Levine, Peter G. *Stronger After Stroke: Your Roadmap to Recovery,* 2nd edition. New York: Demos Health, 2012. Print.

43. Levy, David and Joel Kilpatrick. *Gray Matter: A Neurosurgeon Discovers the Power of Prayer ... One Patient at a Time.* Highlands Ranch, CO: Tyndale House Publishers, 2011. Print.

44. Lewis, Casey. "The Number One Relationship Problem, According to Therapists." *Self Magazine.* 6 May 2015. Web. *www.self.com/story/ marriage-bootcamp-the-number-one- relationship-problem-according-to- therapists.*

45. Lipton, Bruce. *The Biology of Belief: Unleashing the Power of Consciousness, Matter, & Miracles.* Santa Rosa, CA: Elite Books, 2005. Print.

46. Malaspina, Dolores. Personal Interview. 18 October 2018.

47. McCraty, Rollin. *Issues of the Heart: The Neuropsychotherapist.* Eds. M. Dahlitz and G. Hall. Brisbane, Australia: Dahlitz Media, 2015. Print.

48. Moawad, Heidi. "Can Sexual Activity Cause a Stroke?" *Very Well Health.* Reviewed by Richard N. Fogoros, MD. Web. Updated August 25, 2018. *www.verywellhealth.com/sex-and-stroke-3146050.*

49. "More about Recovery of Function and Rehabilitation." *Anat Baniel Method.* 2017. Web. *www.anatbanielmethod.com/adults/ recovery-of-function/more-about-recovery-of-function.*

50. Newberg, Andrew, and Mark Robert Waldman. *Words Can Change Your Brain: 12 Conversation Strategies to Build Trust, Resolve Conflicts, and Increase Intimacy.* New York: Avery, 2012. Print.

51. "The Nine Essentials." *Anat Baniel Method.* 2017. Web. *www. anatbanielmethod.com/about- abm/the-nine-essentials.*

52. Nobel, Jeremy. "UnLonely Overview." *The UnLonely Project.* The Foundation for Art & Healing. 2018. Web. *https://artandhealing.org/ unlonely-overview/.*

53. Norton, Andrea, et al. "Melodic intonation therapy: shared insights on how it is done and why it might help" *Annals of the New York Academy of Sciences* 1169 (2009): 431-6. Print.

54. Ortner, Nick. *The Tapping Solution: A Revolutionary System for Stress-Free Living.* Carlsbad, CA: Hay House, 2013. Print

55. "Preventing Another Stroke." *National Stroke Association.* Web. *www. stroke.org/we-can-help/ survivors/stroke-recovery/first-steps-recovery/ preventing-another-stroke.*

56. Ravn, Karen. "Don't just sit there. Really." *Los Angeles Times.* 25 May 2013. Web. *http://articles.latimes.com/2013/may/25/health/ la-he-dont-sit-20130525.*

57. Rymer, R. "What You Hear Under Anesthesia." *Hippocrates.* May/June 1987: 100-102. Print.

58. Scalisi, Kait. "The Power of Appreciation (Hint: It's Great Foreplay)." *Passion by Kait.* 2018. Web. *www.passionbykait.com/ the-power-of-appreciation-hint-its-great-foreplay.*

59. Schumm, Tom. "The Gift of Brain Cancer." *Chicken Soup for the Soul: Think Positive: 101 Inspirational Stories about Counting Your Blessings and Having a Positive Attitude.* Eds. Jack Canfield, Mark V. Hansen, Amy Newmark. New York: Chicken Soup for the Soul, 2010. Print.

60. "Stroke Facts." *Centers for Disease Control.* 6 Sept. 2017. Web. *www.cdc. gov/stroke/facts.htm.*

61. "Understanding Stroke Risk." *American Stroke Association.* 2014. Web. *www.strokeassociation.org/idc/groups/stroke-public/@wcm/@hcm/@sta/ documents/downloadable/ucm_463745.pdf*

62. "Vision." *National Stroke Association.* 2018. Web. *www.stroke.org/we-can-help/survivors/ stroke-recovery/post-stroke-conditions/physical/vision.*

63. Wasserman Petter, Ilyse. Personal Interview. 21 October 2018.

64. West, Peter. "Sleep May Be Essential for Long-Term Memory." *ABC News.* 25 June 2009. Web. *https://abcnews.go.com/Health/Healthday/ story?id=7921152&page=1.*

65. "What is TIA?" *National Stroke Association.* Web. *www.stroke.org/ understand-stroke/what-stroke/what-tia.*

66. Wood, David. "Every Master was Once a Disaster." *The Kickass Life Podcast.* Ep. 026. Web. *www.thekickasslife.com/ podcasts/026-every-master-was-once-a-disaster/.*

SUGGESTED READINGS

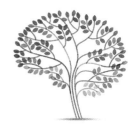

1. *Ask and It is Given: Learning to Manifest Your Desires,* Esther Hicks and Jerry Hicks. Hay House, 2004.

2. *The Biology of Belief: Unleashing the Power of Consciousness, Matter, & Miracles,* Bruce Lipton, Ph. D. Elite Books, 2005.

3. *The Brain That Changes Itself: Stories of Personal Triumph from the Frontiers of Brain Science,* Norman Doidge, M.D. Penguin Books, 2007.

4. *The Brain's Way of Healing: Remarkable Discoveries and Recoveries from the Frontiers of Neuroplasticity,* Norman Doidge, M.D. Penguin Books, 2015.

5. *Chicken Soup for the Soul: Think Positive: 101 Inspirational Stories about Counting Your Blessings and Having a Positive Attitude,* Jack Canfield and Mark Victor Hansen. Chicken Soup for the Soul, 2010.

6. *Conquering Stroke: How I Fought My Way Back and How You Can Too,* Valerie Greene. Wiley, 2008.

7. *The EFT Manual,* 3rd edition, Dawson Church, Ph.D. Energy Psychology Press, 2013.

8. *The Genie In Your Genes: Epigenetic Medicine and the New Biology of Invention,* 2nd edition, Dawson Church, Ph. D. Energy Psychology Press, 2009.

9. *Gray Matter: A Neurosurgeon Discovers the Power of Prayer ... One Patient at a Time,* David Levy, M.D., and Joel Kilpatrick. Tyndale House, 2011.

10. *Love, Medicine and Miracles,* Bernie Siegel, M.D. William Morrow, 1988.

11. *Man's Search for Meaning,* Viktor Frankl. Beacon Press, 2006.

12. *Mind to Matter: The Astonishing Science of How Your Brain Creates Material Reality,* Dawson Church, Ph.D. Hay House, 2018.

13. *My Stroke of Insight: A Brain Scientist's Personal Journey,,* Jill Bolte Taylor, Ph.D. Penguin Books, 2006.

14. *Paralyzed but Not Powerless: Kate's Journey Revisited,* 2nd edition, Kate Adamson. Nosmada Press, 2008.

15. *The Power to Shape Your Destiny: Seven Strategies for Massive Results,* Anthony Robbins (Audio program). Simon & Schuster Audio, 2012.

16. *Stronger After Stroke: Your Roadmap to Recovery,* 2nd edition, Peter G. Levine. Demos Health, 2012.

17. *The Tapping Solution: A Revolutionary System for Stress-Free Living,* Nick Ortner. Hay House, 2013.

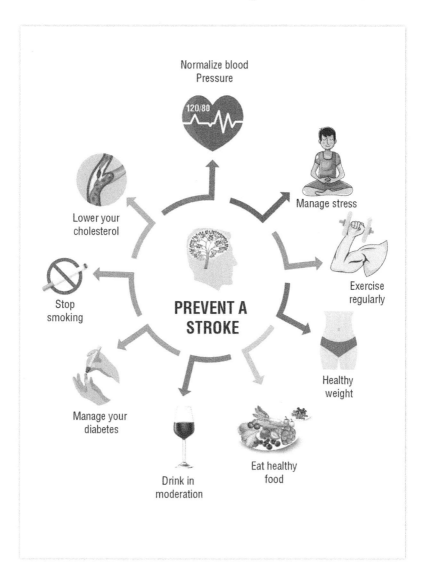

Normalize blood Pressure

Manage stress

Lower your cholesterol

Stop smoking

Exercise regularly

PREVENT A STROKE

Healthy weight

Manage your diabetes

Eat healthy food

Drink in moderation

Made in the USA
Middletown, DE
29 September 2021

49350987R00195